Innovations in Intercarpal Ligament Repair and Reconstruction

Editor

MARCO RIZZO

HAND CLINICS

www.hand.theclinics.com

Consulting Editor
KEVIN C. CHUNG

August 2015 • Volume 31 • Number 3

ELSEVIER

1600 John F. Kennedy Boulevard • Suite 1800 • Philadelphia, Pennsylvania, 19103-2899

http://www.theclinics.com

HAND CLINICS Volume 31, Number 3
August 2015 ISSN 0749-0712, ISBN-13: 978-0-323-39680-6

Editor: Jennifer Flynn-Briggs
Developmental Editor: Colleen Viola

Hand Clinics (ISSN 0749-0712) is published quarterly by Elsevier Inc., 360 Park Avenue South, New York, NY 10010-1710. Months of publication are February, May, August, and November. Business and Editorial Offices: 1600 John F. Kennedy Blvd., Ste. 1800, Philadelphia, PA 19103-2899. Customer Service Office: 3251 Riverport Lane, Maryland Heights, MO 63043. Periodicals postage paid at New York, NY and at additional mailing offices. Subscription price is $390.00 per year (domestic individuals), $606.00 per year (domestic institutions), $194.00 per year (domestic students/residents), $445.00 per year (Canadian individuals), $691.00 per year (Canadian institutions), $530.00 per year (international individuals), $691.00 per year (international institutions), and $256.00 per year (international and Canadian students/residents). Foreign air speed delivery is included in all *Clinics* subscription prices. All prices are subject to change without notice. **POSTMASTER:** Send address changes to *Hand Clinics*, Elsevier Health Sciences Division, Subscription Customer Service, 3251 Riverport Lane, Maryland Heights, MO 63043. Customer Service (orders, claims, online, change of address): Elsevier Health Sciences Division, Subscription **Customer Service, 3251 Riverport Lane, Maryland Heights, MO 63043. Tel: 1-800-654-2452 (U.S. and Canada); 314-447-8871 (outside U.S. and Canada). Fax: 314-447-8029. E-mail: journalscustomerservice-usa@elsevier.com (for print support); journalsonlinesupport-usa@elsevier.com (for online support).**

Reprints. For copies of 100 or more of articles in this publication, please contact the Commercial Reprints Department, Elsevier Inc., 360 Park Avenue South, New York, New York 10010-1710. Tel.: 212-633-3874; Fax: 212-633-3820; E-mail: reprints@elsevier.com.

Hand Clinics is covered in *MEDLINE/PubMed (Index Medicus), Current Contents/Clinical Medicine, EMBASE/Excerpta Medica,* and *ISI/BIOMED.*

Contributors

CONSULTING EDITOR

KEVIN C. CHUNG, MD, MS
Charles B. G. de Nancrede Professor of
Surgery, Professor of Plastic Surgery and
Orthopaedic Surgery, Chief of Hand Surgery,
University of Michigan Health System,
Assistant Dean for Faculty Affairs, Associate
Director of Global REACH, University of
Michigan Medical School, Ann Arbor, Michigan

EDITOR

MARCO RIZZO, MD
Professor, Department of Orthopedic Surgery,
Mayo Clinic, Rochester, Minnesota

AUTHORS

JOSHUA M. ADKINSON, MD
Assistant Professor, Section of Plastic Surgery,
Department of Surgery, Northwestern
University Feinberg School of Medicine,
Chicago, Illinois

JOHN M. BEDNAR, MD
Clinical Associate Professor Orthopaedic
Surgery, Department of Orthopaedic Surgery,
The Philadelphia Hand Center, Thomas
Jefferson University Hospital, Philadelphia,
Pennsylvania

ODED BEN AMOTZ, MD
Research Fellow, Department of Plastic
Surgery, University of Texas Southwestern
Medical Center at Dallas, Dallas, Texas

DAVID J. BOZENTKA, MD
Chief, Hand Surgery; Associate Professor,
Department of Orthopaedic Surgery, University
of Pennsylvania, Philadelphia, Pennsylvania

JOHN T. CAPO, MD
Chief of Hand Surgery, Jersey City Medical
Center, Jersey City, New Jersey; Professor of

Orthopedic Surgery, New York University
School of Medicine, Director of Research
Division of Hand Surgery, NYU Hospital for
Joint Diseases, New York University School of
Medicine, New York, New York

KEVIN C. CHUNG, MD, MS
Charles B. G. de Nancrede Professor of
Surgery, Professor of Plastic Surgery and
Orthopaedic Surgery, Chief of Hand Surgery,
University of Michigan Health System,
Assistant Dean for Faculty Affairs, Associate
Director of Global REACH, University of
Michigan Medical School, Ann Arbor, Michigan

JASON W. DAHL, MD
Fellow, Department of Orthopaedics and
Sports Medicine, University of Washington
Medical Center, Seattle, Washington

MIHIR J. DESAI, MD
Hand, Upper Extremity, and Microvascular
Surgery Fellow, Department of Orthopaedic
Surgery, Duke University, Durham, North
Carolina

JOHN C. ELFAR, MD
Department of Orthopaedic Surgery, University of Rochester Medical Center, Rochester, New York

BASSEM T. ELHASSAN, MD
Associate Professor, Department of Orthopedic Surgery, Mayo Clinic, Rochester, Minnesota

JERRY I. HUANG, MD
Assistant Professor, Department of Orthopaedics and Sports Medicine, University of Washington Medical Center, Seattle, Washington

ROBIN N. KAMAL, MD
Department of Orthopaedic Surgery, Stanford University, Redwood City, California

DANIEL J. LEE, MD
Department of Orthopaedic Surgery, University of Rochester Medical Center, Rochester, New York

STEVE K. LEE, MD
Hospital for Special Surgery, Hand and Upper Extremity Service, New York, New York

DAVID M. LICHTMAN, MD
Department of Orthopaedic Surgery, University of North Texas Health Science Center, John Peter Smith Hospital Network, Fort Worth, Texas

BRETT F. MICHELOTTI, MD
Fellow, Section of Plastic Surgery, Department of Surgery, University of Michigan Health System, Ann Arbor, Michigan

BRYAN W. MING, MD
Department of Orthopaedic Surgery, University of North Texas Health Science Center, John Peter Smith Hospital Network, Fort Worth, Texas

STEVEN L. MORAN, MD
Division of Plastic Surgery, Mayo Clinic, Rochester, Minnesota

NATHAN T. MORRELL, MD
Department of Orthopedics, Brown University, Providence, Rhode Island

RAGHUVEER C. MUPPAVARAPU, MD
Division of Hand Surgery, NYU Hospital for Joint Diseases, New York University School of Medicine, New York, New York

TIMOTHY NIACARIS, MD, PhD
Department of Orthopaedic Surgery, University of North Texas Health Science Center, John Peter Smith Hospital Network, Fort Worth, Texas

MICHAEL C. NICOSON, MD
Hand and Wrist of Louisville, Louisville, Kentucky

NICHOLAS PULOS, MD
Resident, Department of Orthopaedic Surgery, University of Pennsylvania, Philadelphia, Pennsylvania

MARC J. RICHARD, MD
Department of Orthopaedic Surgery, Duke University, Durham, North Carolina

MARCO RIZZO, MD
Professor, Department of Orthopedic Surgery, Mayo Clinic, Rochester, Minnesota

DOUGLAS M. SAMMER, MD
Associate Professor of Plastic and Orthopedic Surgery, Department of Plastic Surgery, University of Texas Southwestern Medical Center at Dallas, Dallas, Texas

MORGAN M. SWANSTROM, MD
Hospital for Special Surgery, Hand and Upper Extremity Service, New York, New York

ERIC R. WAGNER, MD
Resident, Department of Orthopedic Surgery, Mayo Clinic, Rochester, Minnesota

ARNOLD-PETER C. WEISS, MD
Department of Orthopedics, Brown University, Providence, Rhode Island

Contents

A fundamental understanding of the ligamentous anatomy of the wrist is critical for any physician attempting to treat carpal instability. The anatomy of the wrist is complex, not only because of the number of named structures and their geometry but also because of the inconsistencies in describing these ligaments. The complex anatomy of the wrist is described through a review of the carpal ligaments and their effect on normal carpal motion. Mastery of this topic facilitates the physician's understanding of the patterns of instability that are seen clinically.

Carpal instability is a complex array of maladaptive and posttraumatic conditions that lead to the inability of the wrist to maintain anatomic relationships under normal loads. Many different classification schemes have evolved to explain the mechanistic evolution and pathophysiology of carpal instability, including 2 of the most common malalignment patterns: volar intercalated segment instability and the more common dorsal intercalated segment instability. Recent classifications emphasize the relationships within and between the rows of carpal bones. Future research is likely to unify the disparate paradigms used to describe wrist instability.

Perilunate dislocations and fracture dislocations are the result of an axial load with hyperextension and ulnar deviation of the wrist, combined with intercarpal supination. Prompt treatment of injuries is essential. There is a high rate of missed or incorrect diagnosis. In the past, closed management was recommended. These methods proved to be ineffective. Current research and data show better results with anatomic restoration of carpal alignment and direct ligament repair. A combined dorsal and volar approach is preferred. This article reviews the current literature and discusses the surgical techniques to restore carpal alignment and repair the scapholunate interosseous ligament.

The prevalence of ligamentous injury associated with fractures of the distal radius is reported to be as high as 69% with injury to the scapholunate interosseous ligament and lunotriquetral interosseous ligament occurring in 16% to 40% and 8.5% to 15%, respectively. There is a lack of consensus on which patients should undergo advanced imaging, arthroscopy, and treatment and whether this changes their natural history. Overall, patients with high-grade intercarpal ligament injuries are shown to have longer-term disability and sequelae compared with those with lower-grade injuries. This article reviews the diagnosis and treatment options for these injuries.

 Videos of arthroscopic views of the proximal scapholunate (SL) ligament and dorsal SL ligament; arthroscopic examinations of Geissler SLIL injuries; arthroscopic debridement of a proximal SLIL tear; arthroscopic reduction of SL interval; arthroscopic view of second SL K-wire; and fluoroscopy video of K-wire placement across SL interval accompany this article

Wrist arthroscopy is an effective technique for treating acute scapholunate instability. It allows an accurate assessment of the degree and extent of the ligament injury. Partial injuries are effectively treated with arthroscopic debridement and electrothermal ligament tightening. Complete ligament injuries treated arthroscopically allow direct visualization of the torn ligament and assessment of the degree of scaphoid displacement and rotation. The use of arthroscopy allows a more accurate reduction of the scaphoid and lunate at the time of fixation than can be obtained using just fluoroscopy.

Acute treatment of scapholunate instability is important to prevent future complications of dorsal intercalated segment instability and scapholunate advanced collapse. An understanding of the fundamental normal and abnormal mechanics of this problem is vital. Diagnosis in the acute phase is based on clinical and radiographic findings and treatment focuses on primary scapholunate interosseous ligament repair with a reinforcing dorsal capsulodesis. Suture anchor repair with a modified "double-dorsal" capsulodesis is described. Current data show that open repair is a viable option in the acute setting with most patients demonstrating good to excellent functional, clinical, and radiographic results.

Although the true incidence of scapholunate interosseous ligament (SLIL) injury is unknown, a study found that 35% of cadaveric wrists had some degree of scapholunate tear. Of those wrists with SLIL injury, 29% had evidence of arthrosis. Early recognition and treatment of these injuries can delay or prevent the onset of arthritis. This article details treatment options for SLIL injury across the spectrum of pathology with a particular emphasis on chronic scapholunate repair and reconstruction. New techniques and outcomes data also are presented.

Carpal instability arising from an injury to the scapholunate interosseous ligament (SLIL) is commonly seen and treated by hand surgeons. No technique to this date has proved to provide optimal results for primary repair of acute SLIL tear and the treatment of chronic tears of the SLIL. Recently, attention has shifted toward replacement of the dorsal aspect of the SLIL, which is the most structurally and functionally important aspect of the SLIL. This article describes the indications, surgical technique, postoperative treatment and expected results of the use of a bone-retinaculum-bone autograft procedure in the treatment of scapholunate instability.

Treatment of chronic scapholunate ligament injuries can be challenging. Traditional reconstructive techniques, including varied capsulodeses and tenodeses often yield inconsistent results with loss of reduction and radiographic deterioration. As a result, supplemental hardware fixation has become more popular and may allow more robust stabilization of the scapholunate reconstruction. However, these procedures have complications and few data regarding outcomes are currently available. This article evaluates the role of supplemental fixation in the management of chronic scapholunate instability.

Isolated acute lunotriquetral (LT) injuries are an uncommon diagnosis in hand surgery. Diagnosis is aided by a high index of suspicion when pain is localized over the LT joint. Standard radiographs show typically normal findings, leading to advanced diagnostic investigations, including MRI and wrist arthroscopy. Standard treatment options for acute LT injuries include immobilization, arthroscopy, and direct open LT repair.

Chronic lunotriquetral (LT) injuries are less common than scapholunate ligament injuries and difficult to diagnose. They may be associated with positive ulnar variance. Clinical diagnostic tests elicit pain at the LT interval. Although radiographs are typically normal, MRI and wrist arthroscopy can help confirm the diagnosis. When conservative treatments fail, surgical options include LT ligament reconstruction, LT arthrodesis, and ulnar-shortening osteotomy (in patients with positive ulnar variance).

Midcarpal instability has been well described as a clinical entity but the pathokinematics and pathologic anatomy continue to be poorly understood. This article presents a comprehensive review of the existing knowledge and literature-based evidence for the diagnosis and management of the various entities comprising midcarpal instability. It discusses the limitations of the current understanding of midcarpal instability and proposes new directions for furthering knowledge of the causes and treatment of midcarpal instability and wrist pathomechanics in general.

Wrist ligamentous injuries can be challenging to treat successfully. In some cases the ligament repair or reconstruction fails, resulting in instability and progressive degenerative changes. In other cases the original injury is missed, and the patient presents for the first time with established wrist arthritis. Multiple operations have been devised to treat patients with arthrosis secondary to wrist ligament injuries. This article discusses definitive salvage operations such as intercarpal arthrodeses and proximal row carpectomy, as well as other alternatives such as wrist denervation and radial styloidectomy.

HAND CLINICS

FORTHCOMING ISSUES

November 2015
Management of Elbow Trauma
George S. Athwal, *Editor*

February 2016
Pain Management and Hand Surgery
Catherine Curtin, *Editor*

May 2016
Nerve Repair and Transfers from Hand to Shoulder
Amy M. Moore and Susan E. Mackinnon, *Editors*

August 2016
Tendon Transfers in the Upper Limb
Glenn Gaston, *Editor*

November 2016
Treatment of Mutilating Hand Injuries: An International Perspective
S. Raja Sabapathy, *Editor*

RECENT ISSUES

May 2015
Preventing and Avoiding Complication in Hand Surgery
Kevin C. Chung, *Editor*

February 2015
New Developments in Management of Vascular Pathology of the Upper Extremity
Steven Moran, Karim Bakri and James Higgins, *Editors*

November 2014
Options for Surgical Exposure and Soft Tissue Coverage in Upper Extremity Trauma
Amitava Gupta, *Editor*

August 2014
Health Services Research and Evidence-Based Medicine in Hand Surgery
Jennifer F. Waljee and Kate Nellans, *Editors*

May 2014
Flap Reconstruction of the Traumatized Upper Extremity
Kevin C. Chung, *Editor*

RELATED INTEREST

Clinics in Sports Medicine, January 2015
Sports Hand and Wrist Injuries

THE CLINICS ARE AVAILABLE ONLINE!
Access your subscription at:
www.theclinics.com

HAND CLINICS

Preface
Innovations in Intercarpal Ligament Repair and Reconstruction

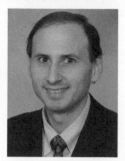

Marco Rizzo, MD

Editor

Intermetacarpal ligament injuries remain a challenging condition to both diagnose and treat for the hand surgeon. Since Drs Linscheid and Dobyns brought the concept of ligament injuries and their sequelae to our attention over 40 years ago, much has been learned about these often difficult problems. The anatomy has been more definitely studied and defined. Mechanisms of injury are better understood. Classification systems are well established for conditions such as scapholunate (SL) dissociation, lunotriquetral (LT) injuries, and midcarpal instability. However, treatments for these conditions remain at times challenging.

The aim of this issue of *Hand Clinics* is to provide an update on the diagnosis and treatment of intercarpal ligament injuries. The introductory articles help to lay the foundation, with Drs Pulos and Bozentka updating us on our current understanding of the anatomy and biomechanics of the intercarpal ligaments. Drs Lee and Elfar follow that with a contemporary review of the injury types, pathomechanics, and injury classification.

Significant acute trauma, such as perilunate and lunate patterns and distal radius fractures, can include intercarpal ligament injuries. Drs Muppavarapu and Capo provide an excellent review of diagnosis and treatment of perilunate injuries. Drs Desai, Kamal, and Richard share their extensive experience and review of the state-of-the-art

for managing intercarpal ligament injuries associated with distal radius fractures.

SL ligament injuries are far and away the most commonly encountered carpal instability pattern recognized and treated by hand surgeons. Five articles are dedicated to the treatment of both acute and chronic injuries. Dr Bednar provides an exceptional review and shares his extensive experience in the arthroscopic management of acute SL injuries, while Drs Swanstrom and Lee provide a thoughtful and thorough outline of open surgical treatment for acute injuries. A variety of treatments for chronic injuries have been utilized. Drs Chung, Michelotti and Adkinson provide a superb review of SL soft tissue ligament reconstruction. Drs Morrell and Weiss share their extensive experience with bone-ligament-bone reconstruction. Finally, there have been significant advances in the use of supplemental stabilization for chronic SL injuries, and Drs Dahl and Huang provide a comprehensive and outstanding update on indications and contemporary use of these techniques and methods.

LT injuries are less common than SL. In addition, they tend to be more subtle in presentation and elusive in diagnosis. A superb review of acute treatment is provided by Drs Nicoson and Moran. Chronic injuries are reviewed by Drs Wagner, Elhassan, and me. Dr Lichtman introduced us to the concept of midcarpal instability, and I feel

Hand Clin 31 (2015) xi–xii
http://dx.doi.org/10.1016/j.hcl.2015.05.001

hand.theclinics.com

fortunate to have him and Drs Niacaris and Ming share the current status of this often difficult problem and their wealth of experience managing the condition.

Finally, arthritis may result in patients with long-standing chronic ligament injuries and instability. Drs Amotz and Sammer provide an excellent review of these patterns of arthritis and current treatment options.

I would like to personally thank all of the authors for their outstanding contributions to this issue of *Hand Clinics*. I sincerely appreciate their efforts and sacrifice. Many thanks to Colleen Viola and Stephanie Wissler from Elsevier for their tireless efforts and assistance in making this issue a reality.

Marco Rizzo, MD
Professor, Department of Orthopedic Surgery
Mayo Clinic
200 First Street Southwest
Rochester, MN 55905, USA

E-mail address:
rizzo.marco@mayo.edu

Carpal Ligament Anatomy and Biomechanics

Nicholas Pulos, MD[a], David J. Bozentka, MD[b],*

KEYWORDS

- Anatomy • Ligaments • Wrist • Carpal

KEY POINTS

- A fundamental understanding of the ligamentous anatomy of the wrist is critical for any physician attempting to treat carpal instability.
- The scapholunate interosseous (SLIO) ligament is the main stabilizer of the scapholunate articulation, providing a flexion moment on the lunate.
- The lunotriquetral interosseous (LTIO) ligament is the main stabilizer of the lunotriquetral articulation, providing an extension moment on the lunate.
- The combined actions of the SLIO and LTIO ligamentous complexes torque-suspend the lunate between the scaphoid and triquetrum.
- Other ligaments may act as secondary stabilizers, whose disruption may increase carpal instability.

INTRODUCTION: LIGAMENTOUS ANATOMY

The anatomy of the wrist was first described in Weitbrecht's illustrations in 1742. Scores of anatomic and kinematic studies have identified the attachments and functions of these ligaments.[1] However, the lack of consistency in describing these ligaments presents a challenge for physicians attempting to understand the ligamentous anatomy of the wrist joint.[2] In addition, the terminology used to describe the ligaments has only recently been standardized.[3]

The bones of the distal carpal row have tendinous attachments but little intercarpal motion as a result of ligamentous and bony constraint. Conversely, the scaphoid, lunate, and triquetrum, which make up the proximal carpal row, have been termed as intercalated segment because of their lack of direct tendinous attachments. The bones of the proximal carpal row move relative to one another by muscular forces extrinsic to the proximal row itself.

The differences between ligaments of the wrist are seen on a histologic scale as well. Hagert and colleagues[4] found that the radial wrist ligaments consisted of densely packed collagen bundles, whereas the dorsal wrist ligament complex contained an abundance of nerves and mechanoreceptors. Thus some ligaments may be more important in providing stability to the carpus, whereas others may serve more proprioceptive functions.

Wrist ligaments can also be described as intracapsular or intra-articular based on their histology. Both types of ligaments are composed of fascicles of densely packed, highly organized parallel collagen fibers. These fascicles are surrounded by perifasicular spaces, which are composed of loose connective tissue containing neurovascular triads. Intra-articular ligaments are covered

No benefits or funds were received in support of this study.

[a] Department of Orthopaedic Surgery, University of Pennsylvania, 3737 Market Street, 6th Floor, Philadelphia, PA 19104, USA; [b] Hand Surgery, Department of Orthopaedic Surgery, University of Pennsylvania, 3737 Market Street, 6th Floor, Philadelphia, PA 19104, USA

* Corresponding author.

E-mail address: david.bozentka@uphs.upenn.edu

entirely by synovial strata, whereas intracapsular ligaments have the synovial stratum only on their deep or joint surface.[5]

This review summarizes the ligamentous attachments to the carpal bones and how they affect normal carpal bone mechanics.

EXTRINSIC CARPAL LIGAMENTS

Extrinsic carpal ligaments connect the forearm bones with the carpus. Because there are no dorsal ligaments between the ulna and carpus, these extrinsic carpal ligaments are divided into 3 groups: palmar radiocarpal ligaments, palmar ulnocarpal ligaments, and dorsal radiocarpal (DRC) ligaments (**Fig. 1**).

In a biomechanical study, Katz and colleagues[6] demonstrated that the palmar capsuloligamentous structures play a more substantial role in preventing both dorsal and palmar carpal translation than the dorsal structures. In their study, the palmar capsuloligamentous structures provided 61% of the restraint to dorsal translation of the carpus and 48% of the restraint to palmar translation.

Palmar Radiocarpal Ligaments

The radioscaphocapitate (RSC) ligament is the most radial of the palmar radial carpal ligaments, originating from the palmar surface of the radial styloid process (**Fig. 2**). According to Berger and Landsmeer,[7] there are 3 major components to this ligament based on the location of insertion. The first component, the so-called radial collateral ligament, is composed of fibers originating from the most distal aspect of the radial styloid process, which course distally to the radiopalmar surface of the waist of the scaphoid. The remaining fibers of the RSC ligament course distally and ulnarly toward the capitate with the radialmost of these fibers inserting into the proximal surface of

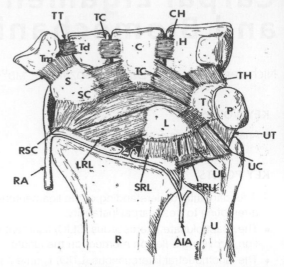

Fig. 2. The palmar carpal ligaments from a palmar perspective. Ligaments: CH, capitohamate; LRL, long radiolunate ligament; PRU, palmar radioulnar; RA, radial artery; AIA, anterior interosseous artery; SC, scaphocapitate; TC, trapezocapitate; TC, triquetrocapitate; TH, triquetrohamate; TT, trapeziotrapezoid; UC, ulnocapitate; UL, ulnolunate; UT, ulnotriquetral. Bones: C, capitate; H, hamate; L, lunate; P, pisiform; R, radius; S, scaphoid; T, triquetrum; Td, trapezoid; Tm, trapezium; U, ulnar. (*From* Berger RA. The ligaments of the wrist. A current overview of anatomy with considerations of their potential functions. Hand Clin 1997;13(1):68; with permission.)

the distal pole of the scaphoid forming the radioscaphoid component. Finally, the fibers of the radiocapitate component, the largest component, interdigitate with fibers of the ulnocapitate (UC) ligament from the triangular fibrocartilage complex (TFCC) just palmar to the head of the capitate.[7] This ligament serves to constrain radiocarpal pronation and ulnocarpal translocation.[8,9] Fibers of the RSC interdigitate with the

Fig. 1. Extrinsic carpal ligaments.

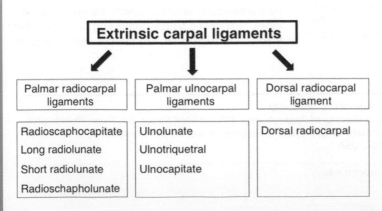

```
              Extrinsic carpal ligaments

     ↙                    ↓                    ↘

┌────────────────┐  ┌────────────────┐  ┌────────────────┐
│ Palmar         │  │ Palmar         │  │ Dorsal         │
│ radiocarpal    │  │ ulnocarpal     │  │ radiocarpal    │
│ ligaments      │  │ ligaments      │  │ ligament       │
└────────────────┘  └────────────────┘  └────────────────┘

┌────────────────┐  ┌────────────────┐  ┌────────────────┐
│ Radioscaphocapitate│ Ulnolunate    │  │ Dorsal radiocarpal│
│ Long radiolunate│  │ Ulnotriquetral │  │                │
│ Short radiolunate│ │ Ulnocapitate   │  │                │
│ Radioscapholunate│ │                │  │                │
└────────────────┘  └────────────────┘  └────────────────┘
```

surrounding ligaments including the UC and tri-quetrocapitate ligaments.[7] This interdigitation can be referred to as the arcuate ligament, deltoid ligament, palmar distal V ligament, or Weitbrecht oblique ligament.[2]

The long radiolunate ligament (LRL) is the central palmar radiocarpal ligament, originating just ulnar to the RSC ligament on the palmar surface of the distal radius. The ligament courses obliquely ulnarly toward the lunate, supporting, but separate from, the palmar aspect of the SLIO ligament.[1,10] Between the RSC and the LRL is the interligamentous sulcus, which represents a weak zone in the wrist capsule, dividing to form the space of Poirier in a perilunate dislocation.[1] The LRL ligament inserts into the radial half of the palmar surface of the lunate and triquetrum.[7] The LRL serves to constrain ulnar and distal translation of the lunate.[9]

The short radiolunate ligament (SRL) as described by Berger and Landsmeer[7] originates just palmar to the lunate facet of the distal radius articular surface. The SRL courses distally to insert as a flat sheet of fibers into the proximal aspect of the palmar surface of the lunate.[7,10] With the LRL and the DRC ligament, the SRL forms the triquetral sling, which functions as a secondary stabilizer of the lunotriquetral interval.[1]

The radioscapholunate ligament is not a true structural ligament, but rather a bundle of connective tissue containing vessels and nerves supplying the SLIO membrane and adjacent osseous structures. This ligament is found in the interval between the LRL and the SRL.[7] The vessels originate from the radial carpal arch, whereas the nerve fibers are terminal branches of the anterior interosseous nerve. Despite being significantly weaker than other ligaments of the wrist, it may serve as a mechanoreceptor for the scapholunate articulation.[1]

Palmar Ulnocarpal Ligaments

Both the ulnolunate (UL) ligament and the ulnotriquetral (UT) ligament, when present,[10] originate from the TFCC, coursing distally to insert onto the anterior surfaces of the lunate and triquetrum, respectively (**Fig. 3**). Berger[1] described the UL, UT, and SRL ligaments all lying in the same plane. The UL ligament is directly contiguous with the SRL ligament forming a proximal V of the palmar floor of the ulnocarpal joint.[1]

The UC ligament originates from a roughened surface at the base of the ulnar styloid, passing distally and superficially to the UT ad UL ligaments before inserting onto the neck of the capitate. Fibers from the UC ligament interdigitate with fibers

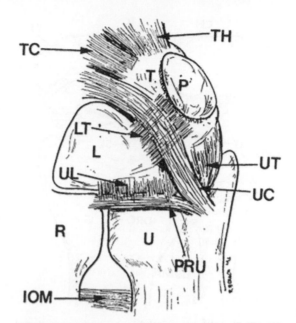

Fig. 3. The palmar ulnocarpal ligament complex from a palmar perspective. Ligaments: IOM, interosseous membrane; LT, lunotriquetral (palmar region); PRU, palmar radioulnar; TC, triquetrocapitate; TH, triquetrohamate. Bones: L, lunate; P, pisiform; R, radius; T, triquetrum; U, ulna. (*From* Berger RA. The ligaments of the wrist. A current overview of anatomy with considerations of their potential functions. Hand Clin 1997;13(1):73; with permission.)

from the RSC ligament forming the arcuate ligament or the distal V.[1,11]

Dorsal Radiocarpal Ligament

The DRC joint is reinforced by only 1 ligament, the DRC ligament (**Fig. 4**). This ligament originates broadly on the ulnar dorsal rim of the distal radius from Lister tubercle to the sigmoid notch and inserts on the dorsal lobe of the triquetrum and lunate, sharing fibers with the dorsal intercarpal (DIC) ligament.[12] The DRC ligament reinforces the dorsal region of the LTIO ligaments, and it serves to constrain ulnocarpal supination and ulnar translation of the carpus.[1]

INTRINSIC CARPAL LIGAMENTS

Intrinsic carpal ligaments originate and insert within the carpus connecting bones of the same carpal row or linking the 2 rows together (**Fig. 5**). A total of 7 ligaments have been identified as crossing over or attaching to the scaphoid or lunate (**Box 1**).[13] However, the SLIO and LTIO ligaments are the primary stabilizers of the proximal row.

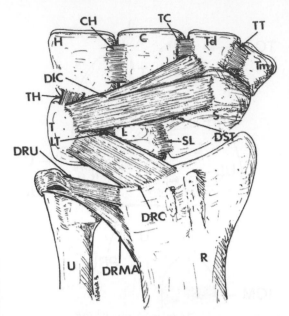

Fig. 4. The dorsal carpal ligaments from a dorsal perspective. Ligaments: CH, capitohamate; DIC, dorsal intercarpal; DRMA, dorsal radial metaphyseal arcuate; DRU, dorsal radioulnar; DST, dorsal scaphotriquetral; LT, lunotriquetral; SL, scapholunate; TC, trapezocapitate; TH, triquetrohamate; TT, trapezoiotrapezoid. Bones: C, capitate; H, hamate; L, lunate; R, radius; S, scaphoid; T, triquetrum; Td, trapezoid; Tm, trapezium; U, ulna. (*From* Berger RA. The ligaments of the wrist. A current overview of anatomy with considerations of their potential functions. Hand Clin 1997;13(1):75; with permission.)

Scapholunate Interosseous Ligaments

The SLIO ligamentous complex is composed of 3 histologically distinct structures forming a smooth connection between the dorsal, proximal, and palmar borders of the scapholunate (SL) articulation. The dorsal SL ligament is a thick, short, transversely oriented collagenous ligament. Distally, it merges to varying degrees with the dorsal scaphotriquetral ligament. Proximally, the dorsal SL ligament merges with a fibrocartilaginous membrane, which contains few superficial longitudinally oriented collagen fibers. The vascular radioscapholunate ligament separates the proximal fibrocartilaginous membrane and palmar SL ligament. Anteriorly, the palmar SL ligament is cartilaginous, but thinner than its dorsal counterpart with more obliquely oriented fibers; it is distinctly separate from the LRL, which lies superficial to it. The distal SL articulation lacks any ligamentous coverage.[14]

A biomechanical study demonstrated the material and constraint properties of the SLIO ligamentous complex. The dorsal SL ligament offered the greatest constraint to translation between the scaphoid and lunate. Both the dorsal and palmar SL ligaments provided significant constraint to rotation. Ultimately, the dorsal SL ligament had the greatest yield strength (260.3 N ± 118.1 N) compared with the palmar SL ligament (117.9 N ± 21.3 N) and the fibrocartilaginous membrane (62.7 N ± 32.2 N). Thus Berger and colleagues[15] concluded that repair of the dorsal SL ligament may provide the greatest likelihood of successfully restoring mechanical integrity between the scaphoid and lunate.

While the SLIO ligamentous complex is the prime stabilizer of the SL joint, the DRC, RSC, DIC, and scaphotrapezial ligaments act as secondary stabilizers. Injury to these secondary stabilizers in the setting of SLIO ligament disruption

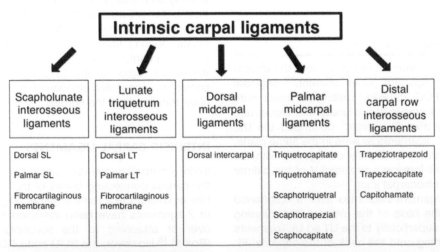

Intrinsic carpal ligaments				
Scapholunate interosseous ligaments	Lunate triquetrum interosseous ligaments	Dorsal midcarpal ligaments	Palmar midcarpal ligaments	Distal carpal row interosseous ligaments
Dorsal SL	Dorsal LT	Dorsal intercarpal	Triquetrocapitate	Trapeziotrapezoid
Palmar SL	Palmar LT		Triquetrohamate	Trapeziocapitate
Fibrocartilaginous membrane	Fibrocartilaginous membrane		Scaphotriquetral	Capitohamate
			Scaphotrapezial	
			Scaphocapitate	

Fig. 5. Intrinsic carpal ligaments. SL, scapholunate.

may lead to further SL instability and altered kinematics.[13,16,17]

Given its course around the scaphoid tuberosity, it was thought that the flexor carpi radialis tendon played a role in carpal stability by causing scaphoid extension.[18] However, in a cadaveric study, Salva-Coll and colleagues[19] demonstrated that this is not the case. When the wrist was loaded, the scaphoid rotated into flexion and supination and the triquetrum rotated into flexion and pronation placing a rotary moment on the proximal carpal row. These opposing moments act to decrease tension on the dorsal SLIO ligament.

Lunotriquetral Interosseous Ligaments

Like the SLIO ligamentous complex, the lunotriquetral (LT) articulation is composed of 3 discrete regions: dorsal, palmar, and a proximal fibrocartilaginous membrane. The thin, proximal subregion provides little constraint to rotation, translation, or distraction of the LT joint. However, in contrast to the SLIO ligamentous complex, which has a relatively thin palmar region and thick dorsal region of obliquely oriented fibers, the LTIO ligamentous complex is thick palmarly with transversely oriented fascicles both dorsally and palmarly. Although both the palmar and volar subregions contribute equally to resist dorsal translation, the palmar subregion resisted 67.3% of palmar translation in a biomechanical study. In terms of rotational stability, the dorsal region is the most important constraint. When Ritt and colleagues[20] selectively sectioned this portion of the LTIO, they found that the total rotation of the LT joint increased by 15.3°.

The combined actions of the SLIO and LTIO ligamentous complexes torque-suspend the lunate between the scaphoid and triquetrum with the SLIO ligaments providing a flexion moment and the LTIO ligaments an extension moment.[21] While sectioning of the dorsal component of the LTIO ligament had little effect on carpal mechanics in a biomechanical study, sectioning of the proximal and palmar subregions produced a volar intercalated segment instability (VISI) pattern with flexion of the lunate and triquetrum.[20]

Although injury to the LTIO ligamentous complex alone results in increased mobility of the triquetrum, it may not lead to collapse.[22] In addition to the LTIO ligaments, secondary stabilizers of the LT joint have been identified on both the volar and dorsal sides of the carpus. Trumble and colleagues[23] identified the ulnar half of the volar arcuate ligament in conjunction with the LTIO ligaments as being important in providing lunate stability against VISI. On the dorsal side of the carpus, the absence of the DRC and DIC ligaments in a biomechanical study allowed the lunate to palmar-flex consistent with a VISI pattern as well. The palmar LTIO, triquetrocaptitate, and triquetrohamate (TH) ligaments were less important in preventing this deformity.[24]

Midcarpal Ligaments

Viegas and colleagues noted that the distal portions of the dorsal SLIO and LTIO ligaments are attached to the DIC ligament. This ligament is the only dorsal midpalmar ligament, originating from the dorsal tubercle of the triquetrum extending radially. This ligament has great variability in its attachments though. It commonly attaches to the dorsal distal aspect of the lunate, inserts into the dorsal groove of the scaphoid, and extends to the dorsal proximal rim of the trapezium, trapezoid, or even capitate in some cases.[25] The DIC ligament is composed distally of thinner fibers extending from the dorsal tubercle of the triquetrum to the dorsal aspect of the trapezoid or capitate and a thicker section extending from the dorsal tubercle of the triquetrum to the dorsal distal aspect of the lunate, dorsal groove of the scaphoid, and proximal rim of the triquetrum.[26]

The DIC serves to stabilize the scaphoid and lunate, preventing dorsal intercalated segment instability.[27] Together with the DRC ligament, the DIC forms a lateral V to create a dorsal radioscaphoid ligament that allows indirect dorsal stability of the proximal pole of scaphoid throughout the range of motion of the wrist.[26]

Palmarly, ligaments connecting the triquetrum to the hamate and capitate form the ulnar arm of the arcuate ligament. The triquetrocapitate ligament originates proximal to the distal edge of the palmar surface of the triquetrum. This ligament courses distally and radially, mirroring the scaphocapitate (SC) ligament to insert into the proximal ulnar half of the palmar cortex of the capitate; it contributes to the ulnar half of the midcarpal joint capsule.[28] The TH ligament originates from the palmar distal edge of the triquetrum, just ulnar to the triquetrocapitate ligament. This ligament courses distally to attach to the palmar surface of the hamate. The TH and triquetrocapitate ligaments are often separated by a sulcus.[28]

Laterally, the palmar scaphotriquetral ligament as described by Sennwald and colleagues[29] spans the midcarpal joint between the distal radial corner of the triquetrum and the distal pole of the scaphoid. Although its attachment to the triquetrum is substantial, its attachment to the scaphoid is thin and fan shaped with fibers interdigitating with those of the RSC ligament.

The SC ligament is a large and stout ligament that originates from the ulnar half of the palmar cortex of the scaphoid and travels obliquely distally and ulnarly to insert on the radial half of the palmar surface of the body of the capitate.[1] The SC ligament forms part of the scaphotrapezium-trapezoid (STT) ligament complex and is an important stabilizer of the midcarpal joint.[18]

The STT ligament complex has 4 components, with the stout radiopalmar scaphotrapezial ligament being the major anatomic stabilizer of the joint (**Box 2**). This ligament originates from the scaphoid tuberosity and inserts along the trapezial ridge. Other components include the palmar capsule, the SC ligament, and the dorsal capsule.[18] In addition to stabilizing the STT joint and scaphoid, the STT ligament may be a secondary stabilizer of the SL articulation.[13]

Distal Carpal Row Interosseous Ligaments

The trapeziotrapezoid (TT) ligaments are composed of both dorsal and palmar regions spanning nearly the entire length of the joint surfaces. The dorsal region forms the floor for the extensor carpi radialis longus tendon and the deep branch of the radial artery.[28]

Box 2
The 4 components of the STT ligament complex

Scaphotrapezial ligament

Scaphocapitate ligament

Palmer capsule

Dorsal capsule

The trapeziocapitate ligaments also consist of dorsal and palmar regions, but unlike the TT ligaments, the insertion is only onto the body and not the head and neck of the capitate. A deep trapeziocapitate ligament has been described, situated entirely within the joint space, lying in a notch on the articulating surfaces.[28]

Similarly, the capitohamate ligament has dorsal, palmar and deep regions. The dorsal and palmar regions span the distal half of the joint, leaving the proximal extension of the pole of the hamate and the head and neck of the capitate devoid of ligamentous connections.

SUMMARY

A fundamental understanding of the ligamentous anatomy of the wrist is critical for any physician attempting to treat carpal instability. Given the anatomic complexity and natural variations, it is not surprising that controversies exist regarding the anatomic descriptions of these ligaments.

A recent systematic review highlights some of the inconsistencies of the various descriptions of scaphoid ligaments. It was found that other than the SC ligament, no ligament has been described consistently.[2] Nevertheless, this it attempts to describe those ligaments of the carpus that have been identified in the literature.

Our knowledge of these ligaments comes from a variety of studies including gross dissections, histologic analysis, biomechanical testing, and more recently 3-dimensional digitization. Our understanding of carpal ligament anatomy will continue to evolve as models of carpal instability in the laboratory continue to drive clinical innovations in intercarpal ligament repair and reconstruction.

REFERENCES

1. Berger RA. The ligaments of the wrist: a current overview of anatomy with considerations of their potential functions. Hand Clin 1997;13:63–82.
2. Buijze GA, Lozano-Calderon SA, Strackee SD, et al. Osseous and ligamentous scaphoid anatomy: part I. A systematic literature review highlighting controversies. J Hand Surg Am 2011;36:1926–35.
3. Gilula LA, Mann FA, Dobyns JH, et al. Wrist terminology as defined by the international wrist investigators workshop (IWIW). J Bone Joint Surg Am 2002;84(suppl 1):1–69.
4. Hagert E, Garcia-Elisa M, Forsgren S, et al. Immunohistochemical analysis of wrist ligament innnervation in relation to their structural composition. J Hand Surg Am 2007;32:30–6.

5. Berger RA, Blair WF. The radioscapholunate ligament: a gross and histologic description. Anat Rec 1984;210:393–405.

6. Katz DA, Green JK, Werner FW, et al. Capsuloligamentous restraints to dorsal and palmar carpal translation. J Hand Surg Am 2003;28:610–4.

7. Berger RA, Landsmeer JM. The palmar radiocarpal ligaments: a study of adult and fetal human wrist joints. J Hand Surg Am 1990;15:847–54.

8. Ritt MJ, Stuart PR, Berglund LJ, et al. Rotational stability of the carpus relative to the forearm. J Hand Surg Am 1995;20:305–11.

9. Viegas SF, Patterson RM, Ward K. Extrinsic wrist ligaments in the pathomechanics of ulnar translation instability. J Hand Surg Am 1995;20:312–8.

10. Nagao S, Patterson RM, Buford WL Jr, et al. Three-dimensional description of ligamentous attachments around the lunate. J Hand Surg Am 2005;30:685–92.

11. Lichtman DM, Wroten ES. Understanding midcarpal instability. J Hand Surg Am 2006;31:491–8.

12. Mizuseki T, Ikuta Y. The dorsal carpal ligaments: their anatomy and function. J Hand Surg Br 1989; 14:91–8.

13. Short WH, Werner FW, Green JK, et al. Biomechanical valuation of the ligamentous stabilizers of the caphoid and lunate: part III. J Hand Surg Am 2007;32:297.

14. Berger RA. The gross and histologic anatomy of the scapholunate interosseous ligament. J Hand Surg Am 1996;21:170–8.

15. Berger RA, Imeada T, Berglud L, et al. Constraint and material properties of the subregions of the scapholunate interosseous ligament. J Hand Surg Am 1999;24:953–62.

16. Short WH, Werner FW, Green JK, et al. Biomechanical evaluation of ligamentous stabilizers of the scaphoid and lunate. J Hand Surg Am 2002;27: 991–1002.

17. Short WH, Werner FW, Green JK, et al. Biomechanical evaluation of the ligamentous stabilizers of the scaphoid and lunate: part II. J Hand Surg 2005;30: 24–34.

18. Drewiany JJ, Palmer AK, Flatt AE. The scaphotrapezial ligament complex: an anatomic and biomechanical study. J Hand Surg Am 1985;10:492–8.

19. Salva-Coll G, Garcia-Elias M, Llusa-Perez M, et al. The role of the flexor carpi radialis muscle in scapholunate instability. J Hand Surg 2011;36:31–6.

20. Ritt MJ, Linscheid RL, Cooney WP, et al. The lunotriquetral joint. Kinematic effects of sequential ligament sectioning, ligament repair, and arthrodesis. J Hand Surg Am 1998;23:432–45.

21. Ritt MJ, Bishop AT, Berger RA, et al. Lunotriquetral ligament properties: a comparison of 3 anatomic subregions. J Hand Surg Am 1998;23:425–31.

22. Viegas SF, Patterson RM, Peterson PD, et al. Ulnar-sided perilunate instability: an anatomic and biomechanic study. J Hand Surg Am 1990;15:268–78.

23. Trumble TE, Bour CJ, Smith RJ, et al. Kinematics of the ulnar carpus related to the volar intercalated segment instability pattern. J Hand Surg Am 1991; 16:355–62.

24. Horii E, Garcia-Elias M, An KN, et al. A kinematic study of luno-triquetral dissociations. J Hand Surg Am 1991;16:355–62.

25. Smith DK. Dorsal carpal ligaments of the wrist: normal appearance on multiplanar reconstruction of three-dimensional Fourier transform MR imaging. AJR Am J Roentgenol 1993;161:119–25.

26. Viegas SF, Yamaguchi S, Boyd NL, et al. The dorsal ligaments of the wrist: anatomy, mechanical properties, and function. J Hand Surg Am 1999; 24:456–68.

27. Mitsuyasu H, Patterson RM, Shah MA, et al. The role of the dorsal intercarpal ligament in dynamic and static scapholunate instability. J Hand Surg Am 2004;29:279–88.

28. Berger RA. The anatomy of the ligaments of the wrist and distal radioulnar joints. Clin Orthop Relat Res 2001;383:32–40.

29. Sennwald GR, Zdravkovic V, Oberlin C. The anatomy of the palmar scaphotriquetral ligament. J Bone Joint Surg Br 1994;76:146–9.

Carpal Ligament Injuries, Pathomechanics, and Classification

Daniel J. Lee, MD, John C. Elfar, MD*

KEYWORDS

- Carpal ligament injuries • Carpal instability • Perilunate instability • Pathomechanics • Classification

KEY POINTS

- Carpal instability is a complex array of maladaptive and posttraumatic conditions that lead to the inability of the wrist to maintain anatomic relationships under normal loads.
- Many different classification schemes have been used to better understand the mechanistic evolution and pathophysiology of carpal instability.
- Progressive perilunate instability describes the global pattern of injury propagation centered on the lunate.
- Two of the most common malalignment patterns are volar intercalated segment instability and the more common dorsal intercalated segment instability.
- Recent classifications have emphasized the relationships within and between the rows of carpal bones, including carpal instability dissociative, carpal instability nondissociative, carpal instability adaptive, and carpal instability complex.

INTRODUCTION

Carpal instability exists when the wrist is unable to maintain its normal alignment as it moves through its motion arc under physiologic loads. Although most carpal instabilities are traumatic in nature, any condition that alters the relationship between the radius, ulna, and carpal bones may result in instability, including inflammatory arthritis, infections, or congenital disorders. Trauma-related carpal derangements may result from simple or accumulated sprains of carpal soft tissue restraints or more severe injury resulting in complete ruptures of the ligamentous stabilizers and dislocation. They comprise a spectrum of injury patterns most commonly incurred as a result of a fall from a standing height, motor vehicle collision, or injury during sporting activities.[1]

Several paradigms have been used to better understand the mechanistic evolution and pathophysiology of carpal instability. Progressive perilunate instability describes the characteristic sequence of injury propagation centered on the lunate. Mayfield and colleagues[2] described 4 stages that progress in an ulnar direction about the lunate (**Fig. 1**). In the first stage, there is disruption through the scapholunate interval. As the distal carpal row is brought into hyperextension, the palmar midcarpal ligaments, in particular the scaphotrapeziotrapezoid (STT) ligament and scaphocapitate ligament, are progressively stretched, pulling the scaphoid into extension and opening the space of Poirier. However, the lunate does not follow the scaphoid into extension because it is tightly constrained by the short and long radiolunate ligaments. The resulting extension force on

Disclosures: The authors have nothing to disclose.
Department of Orthopaedic Surgery, University of Rochester Medical Center, 601 Elmwood Avenue, Box 665, Rochester, NY 14642, USA
* Corresponding author.
E-mail address: openelfar@gmail.com

Hand Clin 31 (2015) 389–398
http://dx.doi.org/10.1016/j.hcl.2015.04.011

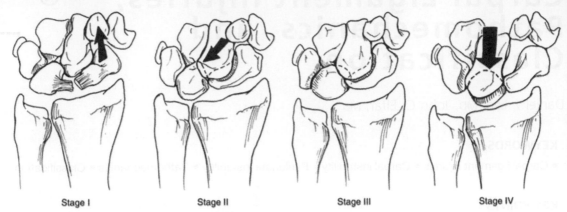

Stage I   Stage II   Stage III   Stage IV

Fig. 1. Stages of progressive perilunar instability. Stage I involves disruption of the scapholunate ligamentous complex (*arrow*). In stage II, the force propagates through the space of Poirier and interrupts the lunocapitate connection (*arrow*). In stage III, the lunotriquetral connection is violated, and the entire carpus separates from the lunate. In stage IV, the lunate dislocates from its fossa into the carpal tunnel, the lunate rotates into the carpal tunnel, and the capitate becomes aligned with the radius (*arrow*). (*From* Kozin SH. Perilunate injuries: diagnosis and treatment. J Am Acad Orthop Surg 1998;6:115; with permission.)

the scaphoid may cause progressive rupture of the scapholunate interosseus ligament (SLIL) in a palmar to dorsal direction.[2,3] If the wrist are instead in radial deviation, then a scaphoid fracture may occur, as opposed to scapholunate dissociation. In the second stage, this force continues on to the space of Poirier, which is located at the palmar aspect of the proximal capitate, lying between the palmar radiocapitate and palmar radiotriquetral ligaments.[3] With progressive wrist extension, the lunocapitate articulation is disrupted as the capitate rotates dorsally relative to the lunate. Further progression of the injury in the third stage violates the lunotriquetral connection, completing the perilunate nature of the injury. The entire carpus separates from the lunate as the lunotriquetral ligaments are torn; the palmar radiotriquetral ligament and ulnotriquetral ligament may also be injured to a variable extent.[3] In addition, in the fourth stage, the dorsal radiocarpal ligament fails, allowing the capitate to reduce from its dorsally displaced position to become realigned with the radius. This realignment causes the lunate to dislocate from its fossa into the carpal tunnel, where it shows a variable degree of rotation.[2,4] Herzberg and colleagues[5] classified perilunate dislocations as stage I injuries and lunate dislocations as stage II injuries. Lunate dislocations are further classified as stage IIA when the lunate shows minor rotation (<90°) and stage IIB when the lunate shows rotation of greater than 90° (**Fig. 2**).

The high-energy traumatic injuries that cause perilunate instability may involve bones, ligaments, or a combination of the two. Injuries that disrupt the scaphoid, capitate, lunate, hamate, or triquetrum bones are termed greater arc injuries.

In contrast, injuries that are confined to ligaments about the lunate (ie, scapholunate, lunotriquetral) are termed lesser arc injuries (**Fig. 3**).[6]

CLASSIFICATION

Various classification schemes have been proposed to aid in the diagnosis and treatment of carpal instability. Two of the most common

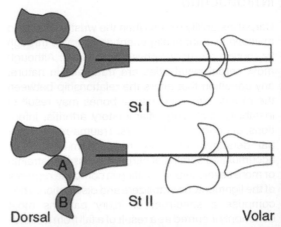

St I

St II

Dorsal   Volar

Fig. 2. Perilunar instability. Stage I (St I) refers to perilunate dislocations with dorsal dislocation on the left and the rarer volar perilunate dislocation on the right. Stage II (St II) refers to lunate dislocations with volar lunate dislocation on the left and the rarer dorsal lunate dislocation on the right. Stage II can be broken down into stage IIA with less than 90° of lunate rotation and stage IIB with greater than 90° of lunate rotation, or enucleation. (*From* Herzberg G. Acute dorsal trans-scaphoid perilunate dislocations: open reduction and internal fixation. Tech Hand Up Extrem Surg 2000;4:3; with permission.)

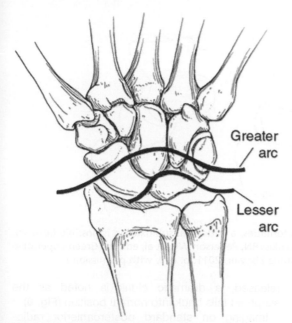

Greater arc

Lesser arc

Fig. 3. The lesser and greater carpal arcs of perilunate instability. (*From* Kozin SH. Perilunate injuries: diagnosis and treatment. J Am Acad Orthop Surg 1998;6:116; with permission.)

malalignment patterns are volar intercalated segment instability (VISI) and the more common dorsal intercalated segment instability (DISI).[7] A VISI deformity describes an abnormal volar tilt of the lunate, typically the result of disruption to the midcarpal stabilizers that results in flexion of the proximal row. A DISI deformity refers to extension of the lunate relative to the capitate and radius and is most commonly observed following rupture of the scapholunate interosseous ligament (**Fig. 4**). Although this nomenclature focuses on the direction of the carpal malalignment, recent classifications have emphasized the relationships within and between the rows of carpal bones. Dobyns and Linscheid[8] described 4 patterns of carpal instability that include the spectrum of intrinsic and extrinsic ligament injuries (**Box 1**). A carpal instability dissociative (CID) pattern occurs when intrinsic ligament injuries cause disruption of bones from the same carpal row.[9] In contrast, a carpal instability nondissociative (CIND) pattern describes injuries to extrinsic ligaments wherein carpal bones of the same row remain linked, but there exists dysfunction between the proximal and distal row or the radius and proximal row.[8,9] In a carpal instability adaptive (CIA) pattern, a derangement outside of the wrist causes the carpal malalignment, most commonly in the setting of a malunion of a distal radius fracture.[10,11] Carpal instability complex (CIC) are instabilities to the

carpus that possess qualities of both CID and CIND patterns.[10]

Carpal Instability Dissociative

Carpal instability that disrupts the bonds between bones of the same carpal row is termed CID.[9] CID may arise from several causes, including scapholunate dissociation (SLD), lunotriquetral dissociation, scaphoid fracture, nonunion, and inflammatory disease. The most common dissociative injuries are discussed here.

Scapholunate dissociation

The term SLD was introduced by Linscheid and colleagues[11] to describe dysfunction in the mechanical linkage between the scaphoid and the lunate with or without malalignment of the carpus. SLD results from a disruption of the scapholunate ligamentous complex, consisting of extrinsic capsular ligaments as well as the SLIL. The SLIL attaches along the dorsal, proximal, and volar margins of the articulating surfaces. The dorsal component has been identified as the strongest and most important stabilizer of the scapholunate interval, because it functions as a primary restraint to distraction, torsion, and translation.[12] The thinner volar component contributes to rotational stability. SLD may progress to rotatory subluxation of the scaphoid when the ligaments secured to both ends of the scaphoid have failed, causing the scaphoid to collapse into flexion and pronation.[13] Although injuries to the scapholunate ligaments may occur in isolation, they may alternatively be the first stage in the process of carpal destabilization around the lunate.

Injuries to the SLIL are among the more common wrist ligament injuries, and approximately 30% of intra-articular distal radius fractures are associated with SLIL injuries.[14,15] These injuries typically occur in the setting of a hyperextended wrist that is in ulnar deviation. As the extended carpus undergoes further loading, the proximal pole of the scaphoid displaces posteriorly while the distal pole displaces anteriorly. Although a complete transection of the SLIL changes the motion between the scaphoid and lunate, it does not result in permanent changes because of the presence of the secondary scaphoid stabilizers, including the palmar radioscaphoid-capitate, scaphoid capitate, and anterolateral STT ligaments.[12] If left untreated, attritional wear to these secondary stabilizers alters carpal mechanics and leads to a DISI deformity as the lunate rotates into abnormal extension and the scaphoid rotates into abnormal flexion. With chronic SLD, the carpus eventually loses congruency, leading to scapholunate advanced collapse (SLAC)

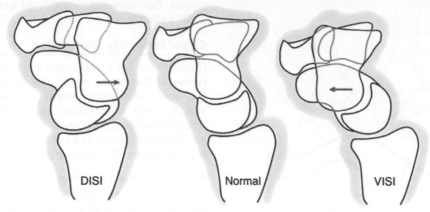

Fig. 4. DISI and VISI deformities of the wrist. In both deformities, a midcarpal subluxation is possible (*arrows*). (*From* Garcia-Elias M. Carpal instability. In: Wolfe SW, Hotchkiss RN, Pederson WC, et al, editors. Green's operative hand surgery. 6th edition Philadelphia: Churchill Livingstone Elsevier; 2011. p. 470; with permission.)

(**Fig. 5**).[13,16] Patients with SLD report a popping or clicking sensation or pain with loading activities. Physical examination reveals tenderness at the dorsal scapholunate interval and pain with wrist extension and radial deviation. In addition, some patients display a positive scaphoid shift test, which is considered diagnostic for SLD.[17] In this maneuver, the examiner applies pressure to the scaphoid tuberosity as the wrist is moved from ulnar to radial deviation. If there is disruption to the SLIL, the proximal pole of the scaphoid subluxates dorsally relative to the radius, causing pain on the dorsoradial aspect of the wrist. As pressure is

released, a dramatic clunk is noted as the scaphoid falls back into normal position (**Fig. 6**).

Imaging on standard posteroanterior radiographs may reveal an increased scapholunate

---

Box 1
Classification of carpal instability

Carpal instability dissociative

1. Scapholunate dissociation

2. Lunotriquetral dissociation

3. Scaphoid fracture

Carpal instability nondissociative

1. Carpal instability nondissociative (CIND)–VISI

2. CIND-DISI

3. Combined CIND

Carpal instability adaptive

Carpal instability complex

1. Dorsal perilunate dislocations (lesser arc injuries)

2. Dorsal perilunate fracture-dislocations (greater arc injuries)

3. Palmar perilunate dislocations

4. Axial dislocations

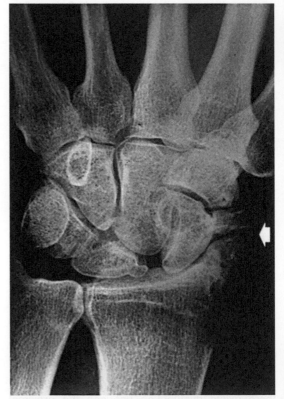

Fig. 5. Example of a SLAC wrist. Osteophyte formation is noted at the radial styloid-scaphoid articulation (*arrow*). (*From* Garcia-Elias M. Carpal instability. In: Wolfe SW, Hotchkiss RN, Pederson WC, et al, editors. Green's operative hand surgery. 6th edition. Philadelphia: Churchill Livingstone Elsevier; 2011. p. 493; with permission.)

(SL) interosseus gap of greater than 5 mm.[14,15] The clenched-fist radiographic view may accentuate the distance seen on unstressed films. In the lateral view, the scaphoid is flexed and the lunate extended in the classic posture of a DISI deformity.[13] A so-called cortical ring sign may be produced by the foreshortened distal pole of the flexed scaphoid (**Fig. 7**).[14] The SL angle is typically greater than 70° (normal 45°–60°), and the radiolunate angle greater than 15° (see **Fig. 7**).

Lunotriquetral dissociation

As with SLD, lunotriquetral dissociation occurs along the spectrum of progressive perilunate dislocation. Relative to the scapholunate ligamentous complex, the triquetrum possesses more extensive ligamentous insertions on its dorsal, ulnar, and palmar surfaces, making lunotriquetral dissociation a more stable injury pattern than SLD. Isolated injuries to the lunotriquetral ligaments may result from a fall onto an outstretched hand with the wrist in extension and radial

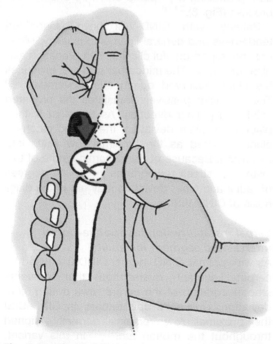

Fig. 6. Scaphoid shift test. Pressure is applied to the scaphoid tuberosity as the wrist is moved from ulnar to radial deviation (*curved arrow*). Disruption to the SLIL causes the proximal pole of the scaphoid to subluxate dorsally relative to the radius (*straight arrow*). As pressure is released, a dramatic clunk is noted as the scaphoid falls back into normal position. (*From* Garcia-Elias M. Carpal instability. In: Wolfe SW, Hotchkiss RN, Pederson WC, et al, editors. Green's operative hand surgery. 6th edition. Philadelphia: Churchill Livingstone Elsevier; 2011. p. 483; with permission.)

deviation.[11] The magnitude of the force is directed onto the hypothenar eminence, causing the pisiform to be driven into the triquetrum, producing its dorsal translation. However, the lunate remains in place as it is restrained volarly by the long radiolunate ligament and dorsally by the distal radius. Displacement of the triquetrum relative to the lunate leads to the accumulation of shear stresses that cause eventual stretching and rupture of the lunotriquetral ligaments.[11,18]

Several investigations have studied the effect of lunotriquetral ligament disruptions on carpal kinematics. In their cadaveric study, Ritt and colleagues[19] observed that sectioning of the palmar lunotriquetral ligament produced divergence of the triquetrum and lunate without carpal malalignment. With additional division of the dorsal radiotriquetral and scaphotriquetral ligaments, the investigators noted a consistent pattern of static carpal collapse into a VISI orientation. These findings are in agreement with previous studies that have shown the palmar lunotriquetral ligament to be the major stabilizer of the lunotriquetral joint as well as the role of the dorsal radiotriquetral and scaphotriquetral ligaments as important secondary restraints.[20,21]

Evaluation of these patients reveals tenderness with ulnar deviation and axial compression. Most patients with lunotriquetral dissociation display a positive lunotriquetral ballottement test as described by Reagan and colleagues.[18] The examiner grasps the lunate between the thumb and index finger of one hand while the triquetrum is translated in a dorsal and volar direction with the fingers of the other hand. Painful shear motion suggests injury to the lunotriquetral ligament.

Standard radiographs may be unremarkable with the exception of possible subtle breaks in Gilula lines. On stress radiographs, there may be increased palmar flexion of the scaphoid and lunate on radial deviation without a concomitant change in the triquetrum, which is suggestive of a loss of the proximal row integrity present in the normal wrist.[20] In the lateral view, the SL angle may be less than 30°, consistent with a VISI deformity.[18] The lunotriquetral angle deviates from its normal mean value of +15° to a mean value of −16°.

Scaphoid fracture

Coordinated motion between the proximal and distal carpal rows depends on the ability of the scaphoid to transfer loads normally. When the integrity of the scaphoid bone is compromised, such as in a fracture, global carpal instability may ensue. The unstable scaphoid fragments displace differently depending on the actions of nearby

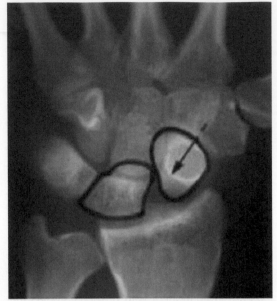

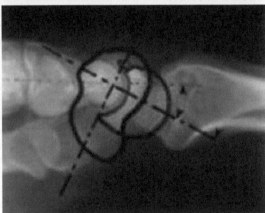

Fig. 7. Posteroanterior (*top*) and lateral (*bottom*) radiographs showing the cortical ring sign (*arrow*) produced by the foreshortened distal pole of the flexed scaphoid and increased scapholunate angle (*arrowheads*). (*From* Walsh JJ. Current status of scapholunate interosseus ligament injuries. J Am Acad Orthop Surg 2002;10:36; with permission.)

structures. Specifically, the distal fragment is loaded into flexion by the trapezoid and trapezium, whereas the proximal fragment moves into extension as it follows the lunate and triquetrum.[22] If left untreated, the resultant nonunion leads to the so-called humpback deformity of the scaphoid, which often leads to a DISI deformity of the wrist.[22,23]

Carpal Instability Nondissociative

CIND is characterized by symptomatic disruption between the radius and the proximal carpal row or the proximal and distal carpal rows, without dysfunction between bones of the same carpal row.[10,11] CIND may be further subdivided into the following groups: palmar CIND or CIND-VISI, dorsal CIND or CIND-DISI, and combined CIND.

Carpal instability nondissociative–volar intercalated segment instability

With ulnar deviation of the wrist, the proximal carpal row rotates from flexion into extension. This movement is aided by the action of the volar midcarpal ligaments, which ensures that the transition occurs smoothly without risk for collapsing into a VISI deformity. Several cadaveric investigations have shown that injury or attenuation to the triquetral-hamate-capitate ligament and scapho-trapezium ligament leads to symptomatic CIND-VISI.[24–26] When these ligaments fail, the proximal row is no longer pulled into extension and instead remains palmar flexed during ulnar deviation. At the same time, there is concurrent volar translation, or volar sag, of the distal row.[24] As the wrist reaches the extreme of ulnar deviation, the proximal row abruptly rotates into an extended position, producing a palpable catch-up clunk in the process (**Fig. 8**).[24,26]

Patients with CIND-VISI have ulnar-sided tenderness and general ligamentous laxity. Many patients report painful clicking with pronation and ulnar deviation. The midcarpal shift test produces the clunk observed during this movement.[25,26] The examiner passively translates the pronated wrist in a palmar direction. As the wrist is then placed into ulnar deviation, the classic catch-up clunk is noted as the proximal row shifts into extension. Because of the dynamic nature of this instability, stress radiographs in varying degrees of radial and ulnar deviation may aid in the diagnosis of CIND-VISI.

Carpal instability nondissociative–dorsal intercalated segment instability

As with palmar CIND, dorsal CIND is caused by carpal ligament dysfunction that prevents smooth rotation of the carpal rows during ulnar deviation. Unlike its counterpart, in CIND-DISI the proximal row remains normally aligned throughout the motion arc.[10,27] In this variant, the clunk occurs from dorsal subluxation of the capitate as the proximal row extends during ulnar deviation. The tendency of the capitate to subluxate dorsally during this movement is likely secondary to insufficiency of the dorsal intercarpal ligament as well as failure of the radioscaphocapitate ligament, which creates excessive laxity in the space of Poirier.[27]

CIND-DISI usually presents in young patients with bilateral hypermobile wrists.[10] They typically

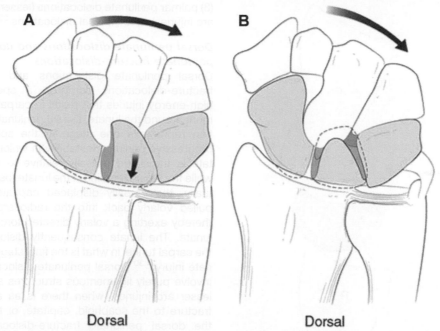

Dorsal   Dorsal

Fig. 8. Pathomechanics of CIND-VISI. (*A*) As the wrist reaches the extreme of ulnar deviation (*large arrow*), the proximal row abruptly rotates into an extended position, producing a palpable catch-up clunk in the process (*small arrow*). (*B*) The lunate assumes an extended posture (*dashed outline*). (*From* Wolfe SW. Carpal instability nondissociative. J Am Acad Orthop Surg 2012;20:578; with permission.)

report pain during grasping maneuvers, particularly when the arm is in supination. The dorsal capitate-displacement apprehension test is useful for diagnosis (**Fig. 9**).[28] The examiner applies dorsal pressure to the scaphoid tubercle while longitudinal traction with flexion and ulnar deviation is applied to the wrist. A painful clunk is noted as the capitate subluxates in a dorsal direction.

Combined carpal instability nondissociative

Combined CIND possesses features of both palmar and dorsal CIND. As in palmar CIND, the proximal row suddenly rotates into extension with ulnar deviation because of attenuation of the volar carpal ligaments. As ulnar deviation continues, dorsal subluxation of the capitate is noted because of additional laxity of the dorsal carpal ligaments.[11] In addition to midcarpal instability, these patients may have radiocarpal instability with abnormal flexion of the proximal row with radial deviation.[10] Combined CIND tends to predominant in young teenagers with global laxity. Examination is often positive for volar carpal sag as well as a positive dorsal displacement test.

Carpal Instability Adaptive

Carpal instability is not always secondary to intracarpal disorder. A CIA pattern occurs when the

dysfunction lies outside the carpus. A classic example of CIA is seen after malunion of a distal radius fracture.[11] The resultant dorsal tilt of the typical malunited distal radius loosens the normally taut palmar midcarpal ligaments, thereby preventing the smooth transition of the proximal row from flexion into extension with ulnar deviation.[10] In most cases, the entire proximal row assumes a flexed posture with dorsal translation of the capitate and distal row.

CIA manifests clinically with clunking or snapping as the wrist is ulnarly deviated along with a lack of range of motion in flexion. Patients may report tenderness to palpation at the midcarpal joint. A history of a distal radius fracture is often given. Standard radiographs show a dorsally malunited distal radius fracture. In the lateral view, the lunate is typically extended and the capitate is variably flexed.

Carpal Instability Complex

Carpal dysfunction that alters the linkage both between bones of the same carpal row (CID) and between carpal rows (CIND) is classified as CIC.[11,29] This pattern of instability may be further subdivided into 4 categories: (1) dorsal perilunate dislocations (lesser arc injuries), (2) dorsal perilunate fracture-dislocations (greater arc injuries),

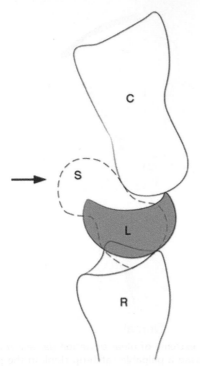

Fig. 9. Dorsal capitate-displacement test. Longitudinal traction with flexion and ulnar deviation is applied to the wrist as dorsal pressure is applied (*arrow*) to the scaphoid tuberosity. The clunk occurs from dorsal subluxation of the capitate as the proximal row extends during ulnar deviation. C, capitate; L, lunate; R, radius; S, scaphoid. (*From* Wolfe SW. Carpal instability nondissociative. J Am Acad Orthop Surg 2012;20:580; with permission.)

(3) palmar perilunate dislocations (lesser or greater arc injuries), and (4) axial dislocations.[29]

Dorsal perilunate dislocations and dorsal perilunate fracture-dislocations

Dorsal perilunate dislocations and perilunate fracture-dislocations comprise a spectrum of high-energy injuries that result in carpal derangement around the lunate. Dorsal perilunate dislocation represents one stage in the spectrum of progressive perilunar instability in which the capitate is translated dorsally relative to the lunate while the lunate remains in the lunate fossa.[4] Eventually, the dorsally displaced capitate may be pulled volarly back into the radiocarpal space, thereby exerting a volarly directed force onto the lunate. The lunate consequently dislocates into the carpal tunnel in what is the final stage of perilunate injury.[4,30] Dorsal perilunate dislocations that involve purely ligamentous structures are termed lesser arc injuries; when there is an associated fracture to the scaphoid, capitate, or triquetrum, the dorsal perilunate fracture-dislocations are referred to as greater arc injuries (**Fig. 10**).[6]

Palmar perilunate dislocations

Palmar perilunate dislocations are infrequent injuries that may follow a lesser or greater arc injury pattern.[31,32] They typically occur in association with dorsally displaced lunate fractures that result in palmar capitate extrusion.

Axial dislocations

Axial dislocations of the carpus generally result from traumatic crush injuries that compress the

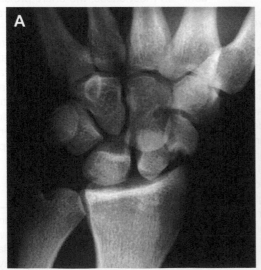

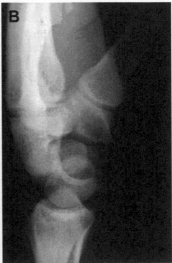

Fig. 10. (*A*) Preoperative posteroanterior and (*B*) lateral radiographs showing trans-scaphoid perilunate fracture-dislocation. (*From* Hildebrand KA, Ross DC, Patterson SD, et al. Dorsal perilunate dislocations and fracture dislocations: questionnaire, clinical, and radiographic evaluation. J Hand Surg Am 2000;25:1071; with permission.)

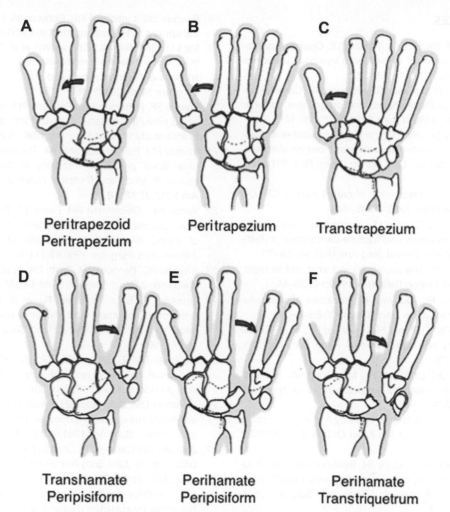

A Peritrapezoid Peritrapezium

B Peritrapezium

C Transtrapezium

D Transhamate Peripisiform

E Perihamate Peripisiform

F Perihamate Transtriquetrum

Fig. 11. Axial dislocations. (*A–C*) In axial radial dislocations, the ulnar column remains reduced relative to the radius, whereas the radial column is displaced (*arrows*). (*D–F*) In axial ulnar dislocations, the radial column remains reduced relative to the radius, whereas the ulnar column is displaced (*arrows*). (*From* Garcia-Elias M, Dobyns JH, Cooney WP III, et al. Traumatic axial dislocations of the carpus. J Hand Surg Am 1989;14:449; with permission.)

wrist in a dorsopalmar direction.[33,34] The high-energy nature of these injuries often causes associated soft tissue compromise and neurovascular injury. In particular, the flexor retinaculum is typically avulsed from its insertions, leading to flattening of the transverse carpal arch. The longitudinally directed force divides the carpus into 2 columns, with 1 column remaining in its reduced position and the other displacing in either a radial or ulnar direction.[34] The direction of the unstable column forms the basis for the 2 major patterns of axial dislocations. In axial ulnar dislocations, the radial column remains reduced relative to the radius while the ulnar column is displaced. In axial radial dislocations, the ulnar column remains reduced relative to the radius while the radial column is displaced (**Fig. 11**).[34]

SUMMARY

Carpal instability is a complex array of maladaptive and posttraumatic conditions that lead to the inability of the wrist to maintain anatomic relationships under normal loads. Many classification schemes have evolved to explain or categorize one or another aspect of this multifactorial condition. An understanding of the anatomy and the general methods of classification is essential to the care of these injuries. Future research is likely to unify the disparate paradigms used to describe wrist instability.

REFERENCES

1. Weil WM, Slade JF III, Trumble TE. Open and arthroscopic treatment of perilunate injuries. Clin Orthop Relat Res 2006;445:120–32.

2. Mayfield JK, Johnson RP, Kilcoyne RK. Carpal dislocations: pathomechanics and progressive perilunar instability. J Hand Surg Am 1980;5:226–41.

3. Kennedy SA, Allan CH. In brief: Mayfield et al. classification: carpal dislocations and progressive perilunar instability. Clin Orthop Relat Res 2012;470: 1243–5.

4. Mayfield JK. Mechanism of carpal injuries. Clin Orthop Relat Res 1980;149:45–54.

5. Herzberg G, Comtet JJ, Linscheid RL, et al. Perilunate dislocations and fracture-dislocations: a multicenter study. J Hand Surg Am 1993;16:768–79.

6. Johnson RP. The acutely injured wrist and its residuals. Clin Orthop Relat Res 1980;149:33–44.

7. Linscheid RL, Dobyns JH. Treatment of scapholunate dissociation. Hand Clin 1992;8:645–52.

8. Wright TW, Dobyns JH, Linscheid RL, et al. Carpal instability non-dissociative. J Hand Surg Br 1994; 19:763–73.

9. Dobyns JH, Linscheid RL, Macksoud WS. Proximal carpal row instability–non dissociative. Orthop Trans 1985;9:574.

10. Wolfe SW, Garcia-Elias M, Kitay A. Carpal instability nondissociative. J Am Acad Orthop Surg 2012;20: 575–85.

11. Linscheid RL, Dobyns JH, Beabout JW, et al. Traumatic instability of the wrist: diagnosis, classification, and pathomechanics. J Bone Joint Surg Am 1972; 54:1612–32.

12. Short WH, Werner FW, Green JK, et al. Biomechanical evaluation of ligamentous stabilizers of the scaphoid and lunate: part III. J Hand Surg Am 2007;32:297–309.

13. Watson H, Ottoni L, Pitts EC, et al. Rotary subluxation of the scaphoid: a spectrum of instability. J Hand Surg Br 1993;18:62–4.

14. Walsh JJ, Berger RA, Cooney WP. Current status of scapholunate interosseous ligament injuries. J Am Acad Orthop Surg 2002;10:32–42.

15. Geissler WB, Freeland AE. Arthroscopic management of intra-articular distal radius fractures. Hand Clin 1999;15:455–65.

16. Watson HK, Ballet FL. The SLAC wrist: scapholunate advanced collapse pattern of degenerative arthritis. J Hand Surg Am 1984;9:358–65.

17. Wolfe SW, Gupta A, Crisco JJ 3rd. Kinematics of the scaphoid shift test. J Hand Surg Am 1997;22: 801–6.

18. Reagan DS, Linscheid RL, Dobyns JH. Lunotriquetral sprains. J Hand Surg Am 1984;9:502–14.

19. Ritt MJ, Linscheid RL, Cooney WP, et al. The lunotriquetral joint: kinematic effects of sequential ligament sectioning, ligament repair, and arthrodesis. J Hand Surg Am 1998;23:432–45.

20. Viegas SF, Patterson RM, Peterson PD, et al. Ulnar-sided perilunate instability: an anatomic and biomechanic study. J Hand Surg Am 1990;15:268–78.

21. Murray PM, Palmer CG, Shin AY. The mechanism of ulnar-sided perilunate instability of the wrist: a cadaveric study and 6 clinical cases. J Hand Surg Am 2012;37:721–8.

22. Vance RM, Gelberman RH, Evans EF. Scaphocapitate fractures: patterns of dislocation, mechanisms of injury, and preliminary results of treatment. J Bone Joint Surg Am 1980;62:271–6.

23. Amadio PC, Berquist TH, Smith DK, et al. Scaphoid malunion. J Hand Surg Am 1989;14:679–87.

24. Trumble TE, Bour CJ, Smith RJ, et al. Intercarpal arthrodesis for static and dynamic volar intercalated segment instability. J Hand Surg Am 1988; 13:384–90.

25. Lichtman DM, Bruckner JD, Culp RW, et al. Palmar midcarpal instability: result of surgical reconstruction. J Hand Surg Am 1993;18:307–15.

26. Lichtman DM, Schneider JR, Swafford AR, et al. Ulnar midcarpal instability-clinical and laboratory analysis. J Hand Surg Am 1981;6:515–23.

27. Johnson RP, Carrera GF. Chronic capitolunate instability. J Bone Joint Surg Am 1986;68:1164–76.

28. Louis DS, Hankin FM, Greene TL, et al. Central carpal instability-capitate lunate instability pattern: diagnosis by dynamic displacement. Orthopaedics 1984;7:1693–6.

29. Green DP, O'Brien ET. Classification and management of carpal dislocations. Clin Orthop Relat Res 1980;149:55–72.

30. Stanbury SJ, Elfar JC. Perilunate dislocation and perilunate fracture-dislocation. J Am Acad Orthop Surg 2011;19:554–62.

31. Conway WF, Gilula LA, Manske PR, et al. Translunate, palmar perilunate fracture-subluxation of the wrist. J Hand Surg Am 1989;14:635–9.

32. Masmejean EH, Romano SJ, Saffar PH. Palmar perilunate fracture-dislocation of the carpus. J Hand Surg Br 1998;23:264–5.

33. Garcia-Elias M, Dobyns JH, Cooney WP III, et al. Traumatic axial dislocations of the carpus. J Hand Surg Am 1989;14:446–57.

34. Reinsmith LE, Garcia-Elias M, Gilula LA. Traumatic axial dislocation injuries of the wrist. Radiology 2013;267:680–9.

Perilunate Dislocations and Fracture Dislocations

Raghuveer C. Muppavarapu, MD, John T. Capo, MD*

KEYWORDS

- Perilunate injury • Lunate dislocation • Wrist instability • Carpal dislocation • Carpal ligament injury

KEY POINTS

- Perilunate dislocations are infrequent injuries often missed on initial evaluation; diagnosis and treatment of these injuries is imperative to restore functional wrist motion and minimize wrist pain.
- Early treatment is necessary to prevent chronic carpal instability and lessen the chance of eventual posttraumatic arthrosis associated with missed or inappropriately treated injuries.
- Open reduction and internal fixation is the treatment of choice for restoring carpal alignment; 3 surgical approaches can be used: volar, dorsal, and combined dorsal–volar approach.
- The goal of proper treatment is a stable wrist with minimal pain and a functional range of motion.
- Most patients will not likely regain normal wrist motion or grip strength, but should have a functional extremity with minimal pain.

INTRODUCTION
Nature of the Problem

Perilunate dislocations are relatively infrequent injuries that are often missed on initial evaluation and involve approximately 7% of all injuries of the carpus.[1–4] These injuries often result from high-energy trauma, including motor vehicle accidents, falls from a height, or contact sporting activities. Owing to the mechanism of injury, patients often present with significant trauma to other organ systems and extremities. Correct diagnosis and treatment of these injuries is imperative to restore functional wrist motion and minimize wrist pain. Early treatment of perilunate injuries is necessary to prevent the devastating complications of chronic carpal instability and lessen the chance of eventual posttraumatic arthrosis associated from missed or inappropriately treated injuries.[5–7]

Patients with unreduced or missed injuries may present many weeks to years after the injury. Although some of these cases may have reasonable function, patients usually present with pain, swelling, possible carpal tunnel syndrome, and flexor tendon ruptures.[5]

Mechanism of Injury

The mechanism of perilunate dislocations was described by a cadaveric study in 1980 by Mayfield and colleagues.[8] The study showed that the application of an axial load causing a hyperextension and ulnar deviation of the wrist, along with intercarpal supination, reproduced a spectrum of injury termed "progressive perilunar instability." Four stages of perilunate injuries were described as the orientation of the carpus is disrupted around the lunate (**Fig. 1**). The pattern of sequential failure begins radially and is transmitted either through the body of the scaphoid (producing a transscaphoid fracture) or through the scapholunate (SL) ligament interval (producing an SL dissociation). The force then propagates to the mid carpal and then ulnar aspects of the wrist. Other variants include transradial styloid and scaphocapitate injury patterns.

Classification

- Stage I: disruption of the SL and radioscapho-capitate ligaments.

Division of Hand Surgery, NYU Hospital for Joint Diseases, New York University School of Medicine, 530 First Avenue, Suite 8U, New York, NY 10016, USA
* Corresponding author.
E-mail address: njhanddoc@yahoo.com

Hand Clin 31 (2015) 399–408
http://dx.doi.org/10.1016/j.hcl.2015.04.002
0749-0712/15/$ – see front matter © 2015 Elsevier Inc. All rights reserved.

hand.theclinics.com

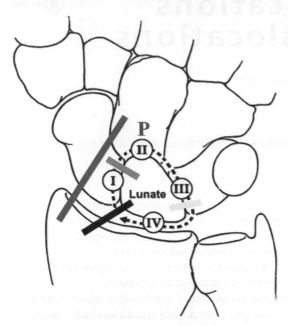

Fig. 1. Pattern and progression of perilunate injury. Radioscaphocapitate ligament (*red line*), Radiolunate ligament (*black line*), Scapholunate ligament (*green line*), Lunotriquetral ligament (*yellow line*). (*Courtesy of* John T. Capo, MD, New York, NY.)

- Stage II: disruption of the lunocapitate association.
- Stage III: failure of the lunotriquetral interosseous ligament and lunotriquetral ligament. The entire carpus in essence separates from the lunate and is usually dislocated dorsally.
- Stage IV: palmar lunate dislocation into the carpal tunnel. The remaining carpus often self-reduces on the radius and does not seem to be dislocated.

Mayfield and associates demonstrated that slower application of load produced the fracture variants (radial styloid, scaphoid, and/or capitate) before the lunate dislocation and termed these as "greater arc injuries." A more rapidly applied force produced purely ligamentous disruptions, termed as "lesser arc injuries."[8]

Presentation

The typical presentation of an acute perilunate dislocation includes pain and swelling about the wrist. There is a true spectrum of perilunate injuries ranging from those caused by low-energy to high-energy mechanisms.[4] In low-energy patterns, the deformity may be more subtle than expected with no associated nerve or tendon injuries.[7] In a lunate dislocation, the lunate can come to lie within the carpal tunnel. Performing a thorough neurovascular assessment of the upper extremity is important. Obtaining and interpreting true biplane radiographs is essential to making an accurate diagnosis.

- The posteroanterior view shows disruption of the normal carpal arcs (Gilula's arcs; **Fig. 2**).
- Gilula's 3 arcs are formed by the proximal and distal articular surfaces of the proximal carpal row, and the proximal cortical margins of capitate and hamate.[9]
- The lateral radiograph reveals loss of colinearity between the capitate, lunate, and the radius (**Fig. 3**). Most often, the distal carpal row is dislocated dorsally or there is a large dorsal intercalated segment instability deformity.
- Traction radiographs can be used to further assess the injury pattern, if there is significant overlap of the carpal bones or difficulty with evaluating the images.
- CT is helpful if there are complex associated fractures, such as a scaphoid or triquetral fracture. These higher level imaging studies should be done after closed reduction.[7]

Closed Reduction

- Initial treatment consists of immediate closed manipulation to achieve reduction and immobilization. This also reduces pressure on the soft tissue and median nerve.

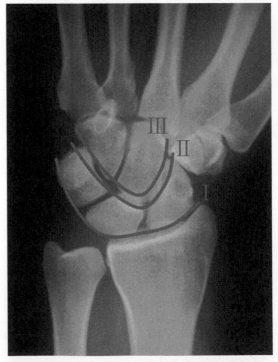

Fig. 2. Posteroanterior radiograph showing the Gilula's arcs. Radioscaphocapitate ligament (*red line*). (*Courtesy of* John T. Capo, MD, New York, NY.)

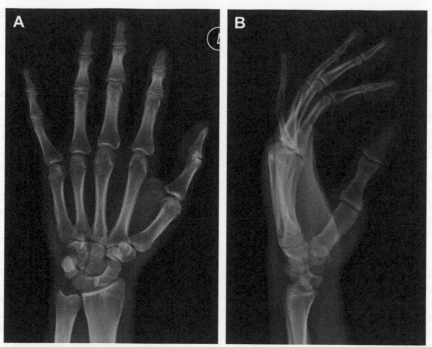

Fig. 3. (*A, B*) Posteroanterior and lateral radiograph of a stage III perilunate dislocation. The lunate is shown in a flexed position with dislocation of the lunocapitate articulation. The lunate is still in the lunate fossa but there is an absence of alignment between the radius, lunate, and capitate. (*Courtesy of* John T. Capo, MD, New York, NY.)

- Reduction is usually undertaken with the patient under intravenous sedation.
- The arm is suspended in longitudinal traction.
- With the wrist extended and maintaining traction, the surgeon's thumb is placed volarly against the lunate and is used to apply a dorsally directed force to push the lunate back into its fossa.
- The wrist is brought progressively into flexion, maintaining the dorsally directed force against the lunate.[4]
- Failure to achieve a reduction via closed means often indicates interposed volar capsule and necessitates an open procedure.[10–12]

TREATMENT OPTIONS

Closed reduction and immobilization has been the historical gold standard treatment for perilunate injuries.[13] The current consensus is that anatomic restoration of the carpus is difficult to achieve and maintain via nonoperative means.[3,6] Multiple studies have shown that the complex intercarpal relationships are maintained poorly by means of closed reduction and immobilization alone.[13,14] The "paradox of reduction" has been coined to describe this difficulty in closed reduction. For closure of the SL gap radial deviation is needed,

but for correction of the scaphoid flexion, ulnar deviation is required. Studies comparing perilunate injuries treated conservatively versus those that underwent open treatment have shown consistently better results in those patients that underwent operative fixation.[3,5,10–12]

Apergis and colleagues[14] used a scoring system based on pain, occupation, range of motion, and grip strength to compare the results of conservative versus surgical repair. The group treated with closed reduction had fair results in 3 and poor results in 5. The group treated surgically (early open reduction) had a better clinical score with 4 excellent, 9 good, and 7 fair or poor results.

Inadequate realignment of the carpal bones in a perilunate dislocation has been shown to be associated with chronic carpal instability, traumatic arthritis with persistent pain, SL advanced collapse, and loss of motion.[4,15] Open reduction permits direct visualization of the injury and allows for restoration of the carpal anatomy.[10] It is for these reasons that open reduction and internal fixation, through a dorsal and volar approach with combined carpal tunnel release, is our preferred method of treatment for all acute perilunate dislocations.

Open perilunate injuries should be considered an orthopedic emergency. Patients should be emergently taken to the operating room for irrigation and debridement, followed by repair of the injured structures. If the physician is on call is not comfortable with complete treatment of the injuries, then irrigation and debridement and carpal tunnel release should be performed. Timely referral to a hand surgeon should occur within the next 24 to 36 hours. The prognosis of closed injuries is better owing to lower magnitude of energy involved and also preservation of soft tissue envelope.[5]

Despite the overall consensus that open reduction and internal fixation is the treatment of choice for restoring carpal alignment, the ideal surgical approach is less explicit.[10–12] There are 3 basic surgical approaches that can be used: volar, dorsal, and a combined dorsal–volar approach.

- The volar or palmar approach is used typically for reduction of the lunate and carpal tunnel release.
- The volar approach also allows the surgeon to complete a direct repair of the capsular tear at the space of Poirier.
- The volar approach can also be used for repair of the volar lunotriquetral ligament and possibly the SL ligament as well. Often there are ostechondral fragments volarly that can be removed.[16]
- The dorsal approach provides exposure of the carpus for restoring alignment and repairing the SL interosseous ligament (SLIL), which is thought to be the key to a successful long-term outcome.[3,9]
- A dorsal approach also allows the surgeon to address any scaphoid and other carpal bone fractures.
- The combined dorsal–volar approach offers the advantages of both and is the preferred choice of the senior author because it allows access to all the injured structures.

There are certain injury patterns that are not managed easily with just open reduction and internal fixation. Associated comminuted distal radius fractures and severe soft tissue injuries or ligament disruption often require spanning external fixation for additional stabilization.[9] Proximal row carpectomy and scaphoid excision with 4-corner fusion are usually reserved for missed or chronic perilunate dislocations.

SURGICAL TECHNIQUE
Preparation and Patient Positioning

- The arm is prepped and draped on a radiolucent hand table with the patient in the supine position.

SURGICAL APPROACH AND PROCEDURE
Volar Approach

- When the lunate is not dislocated volarly, the carpus can be approached first from either the dorsal or volar side.
- If the lunate is dislocated volarly. we approach from the volar side first to facilitate reduction of the lunate.
- An extended carpal tunnel incision is used, commencing 2 to 3 cm proximal to the wrist crease in line with the ulnar border of the palmaris longus tendon.
- The incision is angled ulnarly across the wrist crease to avoid injury to the palmar cutaneous branch of the median nerve. It is then extended along the line of the ring finger ray and ends in the mid palm, at the distal border of the transverse carpal ligament. This extends past Kaplan's cardinal line.
- The transverse carpal ligament and the antebrachial fascia are incised and the carpal tunnel is completely decompressed.
- The flexor tendons along with the median nerve are retracted radially to expose the lunate (**Fig. 4**).
- The lunate is then reduced using the same technique as described for closed manipulation, but in this case with direct pressure on the bone itself.
- Reduction of the lunate can sometimes be impeded by the interposed capsule. If that occurs, the capsule will need to be moved out of the way to allow the lunate to relocate.
- After the reduction, the volar capsular rent and ligamentous complex are repaired with a 3-0 or 4-0 nonabsorbable suture to prevent the lunate from dislocating during the remainder of the operative procedure.

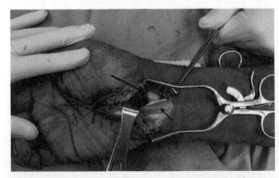

Fig. 4. Volar approach for a perilunate injury. The carpal tunnel has been released. The lunate (large *arrow*) is dislocated and can be visualized in the proximal aspect of the carpal tunnel. The contents of the carpal tunnel (small *arrow*) are being retracted ulnarly. (*Courtesy of* John T. Capo, MD, New York, NY.)

Dorsal Approach

- A moist gauze sponge is placed in the volar wound and the hand and arm are pronated.
- The dorsal approach consists of a 4- to 5-cm longitudinal incision in line with Lister's tubercle.
- Skin flaps are raised radially and ulnarly and the incision is carried down to the extensor retinaculum.
- The retinaculum is divided in line with the third dorsal compartment, and the extensor pollicis longus tendon is identified distally and retracted radially. The third compartment does not have to be completely opened. Only the distal 1 cm is released.
- The second and fourth compartments are then reflected off the dorsal capsule.
- A capsular tear is usually encountered with the dorsal radial carpal ligament being avulsed from the radius.
- A capsulotomy is extended either longitudinally or in a ligament-sparing fashion along the fibers of the dorsal radiocarpal and dorsal intercarpal ligaments (**Fig. 5**).[17]
- The cartilage surfaces of the carpal bones are inspected and an intraoperative assessment of the injury pattern is made.
- Small osteochondral fragments are removed from the joint.
- The joints are irrigated to remove any hematoma and other debris.
- Kirschner wires (K-wires) are placed into the scaphoid and lunate and used as "joy-sticks" to correct the intercalated segment instability pattern. The scaphoid pin is placed at 45° from distal to proximal and the lunate pin in

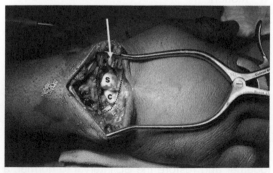

Fig. 5. Dorsal approach for a perilunate injury. There is a tear of the dorsal radiocarpal ligament, which is extended into a "v-flap" capsulotomy (*black dotted line*). A self-retaining retractor is used to retract the capsule (*yellow arrow*). The scaphoid (*S*) and capitate (*C*) are visualized easily. The lunate cannot be visualized because it is dislocated volarly. (*Courtesy of John T. Capo, MD, New York, NY.*)

placed in a proximal to distal orientation at a similar angle.
- The joysticks are used to extend the scaphoid and flex the lunate, which will lead to the SL interval closing. This is done by bringing the scaphoid pin proximal and the lunate pin distal, thus making the pins colinear, and then compressing them together to decrease the SL gap.
- Often the midcarpal and lunotriquetral joints improve with restoration of the normal alignment of the scaphoid and lunate. They often are not reduced completely.
- Once the carpus is in alignment, percutaneous intercarpal pinning is done to maintain the carpal relationship (**Fig. 6**).
- Two K-wires (0.045) are used to stabilize the scaphoid to the lunate. These pins are placed through a small open incision to avoid injury to the extensor tendons of compartments 1, 2, and 3 and the superficial radial nerve.
- The lunotriquetral joint is pinned from the ulnar side of the wrist, percutaneously, starting at a point dorsal to the pisiform and aiming slightly proximal.
- The midcarpal joint is then reduced by placing dorsal to volar pressure on the hand and thus the distal carpal row. This maneuver corrects the dorsal subluxation of the capitate and any remaining dorsal intercalated segment instability deformity.
- Pins are placed from the triquetrum into the hamate and from the scaphoid into the capitate to stabilize the mid carpal joint. The radial-sided pin is used to secure the distal scaphoid to the capitate to help prevent scaphoid flexion.
- Carpal alignment and K-wire positions are confirmed with intraoperative fluoroscopy. The pins are cut to lie under the skin.
- Once the carpus is aligned and stabilized, the SLIL needs to be repaired.
- The ligament is usually avulsed off the dorsal lunate.
- The bony bed is prepared by removing any interposed soft tissue and creating a bleeding surface.
- One or 2 suture anchors are placed into the bed and used to repair the dorsal portion of the ligament (see **Fig. 6**).
- Any osteochondral fragment that may still be attached to the ligament is preserved and incorporated into the repair for better suture retention and healing potential.[18]
- The capsulotomy incision is reapproximated with braided nonabsorbable 3-0 or 4-0 sutures in an interrupted fashion.

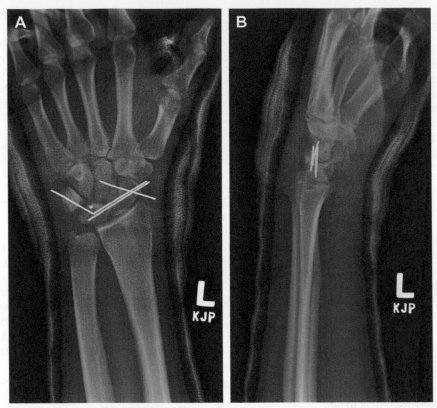

Fig. 6. (*A, B*) Posteroanterior and lateral radiographs showing the appropriate stabilization of the carpus with Kirschner wires (K-wires). Two radiolunate K-wires were used to stabilize the scaphoid to the lunate. Scaphoca-pitate and lunotriquetral K-wires were used to reduce the rest of the carpus. The scapholunate interosseous lig-ament was repaired to the lunate with a suture anchor. (*Courtesy of* John T. Capo, MD, New York, NY.)

- If the dorsal radial carpal ligament has avulsed from the distal radius, it is repaired with a suture anchor placed along the dorsal lip of the radius.
- Then the retinaculum is repaired, leaving the extensor pollicis longus free distally but still within its compartment proximally.
- The skin is closed with nylon sutures.
- A sugar-tong splint is placed with the wrist and forearm in the neutral position.

Immediate Postoperative Care

- Finger motion is started immediately.
- At the first postoperative visit (10–14 days) the sutures are removed and the patient is placed in a long arm cast to immobilize the wrist, fore-arm, and elbow.
- At 3 to 4 weeks postoperatively, the patient is then converted to a Muenster–Spica cast to allow elbow flexion and extension but no pro-nation or supination of the forearm.
- At 6 weeks, the extremity is placed in a short arm thumb Spica cast.

Rehabilitation and Recovery

- The K-wires are removed in the operating room at 10 weeks (**Fig. 7**).
- Therapy is started for wrist and elbow range of motion.

OPERATIVE PEARLS
Difficulty Restoring Carpal Alignment

Sometimes it may be very difficult to restore the normal relationships of the carpal bones. Part of the problem may be that the initial joysticks may not be in the optimal positions. A useful trick is to partially reduce the SL interval, then place a sec-ond set of joysticks in better positions to help com-plete the reduction. To compress the bones together and restore the SL interval to normal, a pointed bone reduction clamp is then placed across the scaphoid and lunate.

The carpus can be highly unstable owing to loss of capsular and ligamentous attachment to the distal radius. In these cases, even with use of the joystick maneuver, the scaphoid and lunate will not assume the normal alignment on the distal

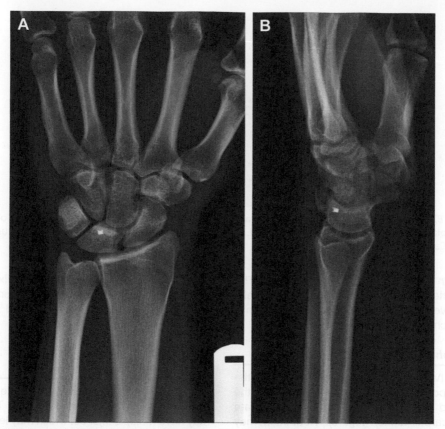

Fig. 7. (*A, B*) Posteroanterior and lateral radiographs at 6 month follow-up with the Kirschner wires (K-wires) removed. The lunate is well-seated in the lunate fossa. Excellent alignment is maintained between the radius, lunate, and capitate. (*Courtesy of* John T. Capo, MD, New York, NY.)

radius simultaneously. It may be necessary to secure provisionally the radiolunate articulation with a K-wire from the radial metaphysis into the lunate. This maneuver will help to stabilize provisionally the important "keystone" of carpus, the radiolunate joint, and will facilitate reduction of the rest of the carpal bones to the now stable lunate.

The radiolunate pin can be removed at the end of the case or left in place to provide additional stability. However, the increased risk of pin loosening, chondrolysis, and broken hardware should be taken into consideration with radiocarpal pinning. If the carpus is highly unstable or if the injury presents at a subacute or chronic time period, an external fixator may be used to help with reduction and then can be left in place for postoperative stabilization.

Irreparable Scapholunate Interosseous Ligament

One of the key steps to a good outcome is reestablishing a stable SL interval. However, often the SLIL is torn in such a way that it cannot be repaired securely. When encountered with this situation, we denude the cartilage from the SL articulation (similar to that described by Rosenwasser and colleagues[19]) to try to promote some stability by chondrodesis. This maneuver is performed before the intercarpal pinning step.

We still advocate trying to repair the remnant SLIL as best as possible, but it is also augmented with a dorsal capsulodesis. A 3- to 5-mm wide capsular flap is fashioned, leaving it attached to the distal pole of the scaphoid. Its proximal end is then sutured to the dorsum of the lunate with suture anchors. By attaching the proximal ligament transfer to the lunate and not the radius, postoperative wrist flexion is not restricted.

Alternatively, the SL interval can be closed down with the reduction and stabilization of the scaphoid and lunate with screws or pins.[19] Ring and colleagues[20] have found that the use of buried screws, compared with pins, has a lower complication rate. Bioabsorbable pins or screws can be used to stabilize across the SL interval but they are less stiff than their stainless steel counterparts. Despite this limitation, the bioabsorbable pins and

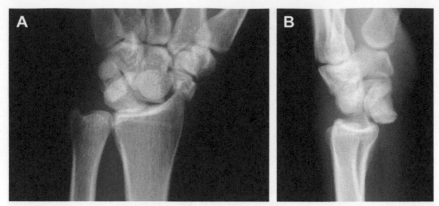

Fig. 8. (*A, B*) Posteroanterior and lateral radiograph of a stage IV transscaphoid perilunate dislocation. The lunate is volarly dislocated into the carpal tunnel. The remaining carpus is aligned with the radius. (*Courtesy of* John T. Capo, MD, New York, NY.)

screws can withstand relatively high loads.[21] The use of buried K-wires left in place for 10 weeks and removed in the operating room has been a reliable technique in our practice.

Transscaphoid Perilunate Dislocation

In stage IV transscaphoid injury patterns, the proximal pole of the scaphoid travels with the lunate and may be dislocated with the lunate into the carpal tunnel (**Fig. 8**). Reduction may require enlarging the rent in the volar capsule. The scaphoid fracture is assessed and reduced through the dorsal capsulotomy. A headless screw is placed, usually from proximal to distal, through the central axis of the bone (**Fig. 9**). Care must be taken not to dissect distally on the scaphoid because this removes the important blood supply that enters on the scaphoid dorsal ridge.

Often the SLIL is attenuated in association with a scaphoid fracture. In such cases, the SL interval is

pinned in addition to the scaphoid fixation. The midcarpal (scaphocapitate) and lunotriquetral pinning is performed as described previously (see **Fig. 9**).

PITFALLS
Delayed Diagnosis

The major pitfall in treating perilunate carpal injuries is delayed or missed diagnosis. The patient may have multiple injuries, which may lead to inadequate workup and diagnostic imaging of the extremity injuries. The diagnosis can also be missed owing to inexperienced personnel interpreting the radiographs. Proper interpretation of radiographs and recognition of the loss of normal arcs of the carpal bones will help to decrease the chances of missed or delayed diagnosis. A perilunate dislocation that has not been identified by 4 weeks after the injury is considered a missed or delayed diagnosis. For patients less than 30 years old, these injuries can still be treated

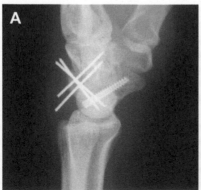
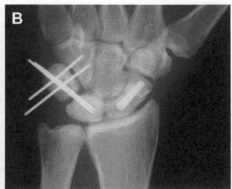

Fig. 9. (*A, B*) Lateral and posterioranterior radiographs showing Kirschner wire (K-wire) stabilization of the carpus. Lunotriquetral and triquetocapitate K-wires were used to reduce the carpus. A screw was used to stabilize the scaphoid fracture. (*Courtesy of* John T. Capo, MD, New York, NY.)

with reduction and reconstruction. For older patients, a missed perilunate dislocation greater than 4 weeks may require a salvage procedure, such as a proximal row carpectomy, owing to difficulty in reduction and poor outcomes associated with reconstruction.

Pin Track Infection and Septic Arthritis

- The pins need to be kept in place for 10 weeks to stabilize the reconstruction and protect the repair.
- Leaving pins outside the skin can avoid an additional trip to the operating room for wire removal, but they are susceptible to infection.
- Superficial pin site infection can spread to the deeper layers and lead to septic arthritis and osteomyelitis.
- Pins should be cut well under the skin to avoid skin irritation from a buried but prominent pin.
- Buried pins also make splint and cast application easier.

SUMMARY

We have changed our treatment strategy for perilunate dislocations as we have come to better understand the mechanism of injury. Operative fixation has become the mainstay of treatment for perilunate injuries. Apergis and colleagues[14] compared the result of closed treatment versus operative repair in patients with perilunate dislocations and illustrated that all patients treated closed had poor results, whereas those treated open with a combined dorsal–volar approach reported good to excellent results.

Herzberg and colleagues[5] showed in their large multicenter study of 166 perilunate dislocations and fracture dislocations that, despite satisfactory clinical outcomes, 56% of patients who were treated surgically had radiographic evidence of arthritis. Fortunately, the presence of arthrosis does not lead predictably to wrist pain. The best results were seen in patients treated early, and a delay in diagnosis was shown to have an adverse effect on the outcome. In a similar study, Hildebrand and colleagues[7] used multiple, validated outcome instruments to assess the results in a cohort of 22 patients who underwent operative fixation of a perilunate injury with a combined dorsal–volar approach at 1-year follow-up. They found that most patients reported decreased grip strength and motion, and had radiographic evidence of arthritis and early carpal collapse. Despite this, 3 out of 4 patients were able to return to full duties in their previous occupations.

Based on a follow-up of 13 years by Forli and colleagues,[22] signs of posttraumatic arthritis increase progressively, but clinically, they were well-tolerated. An accurate articular restoration is an essential step in treatment because carpal malalignment has been recognized as a precursor to joint deterioration. Even with perfect bony alignment and complete ligamentous healing, patients should not expect to have a normal wrist. The goal of proper treatment is a stable wrist with minimal pain and a functional range of motion. The postoperative protocol involves intensive occupational therapy.[23] Athletes should participate in therapy for range of motion and strengthening to guide their return to sports, which may take up to a year.[10]

Perilunate dislocations and fracture dislocations are complex wrist injuries. To achieve a good outcome, the injury must be recognized early and appropriately diagnosed.[23] Treatment should consist of realigning the disrupted carpal articulations and repairing or reconstructing the intercarpal and radiocarpal ligaments.[24] A combined dorsal–volar approach provides the best exposure and allow the surgeon to appropriately reduce and stabilize the injury. An anatomic reduction leads to decreased risk of arthritis; however, most patients will not likely regain normal wrist motion or grip strength, but should have a functional extremity with minimal pain.

REFERENCES

1. Weil WM, Slade JF 3rd, Trumble TE. Open and arthroscopic treatment of perilunate injuries. Clin Orthop Relat Res 2006;445:120–32.
2. Campbell RD Jr, Thompson TC, Lance EM, et al. Indications for open reduction of lunate and perilunate dislocations of the carpal bones. J Bone Joint Surg Am 1965;47:915–37.
3. Moran SL, Ford KS, Wulf CA, et al. Outcomes of dorsal capsulodesis and tenodesis for treatment of scapholunate instability. J Hand Surg Am 2006;31: 1438–46.
4. Garcia-Elias M. Carpal instabilities and dislocations. In: Green D, Hotchkiss R, Pederson W, editors. Green's operative hand surgery, vol. 1, 4th edition. Philadelphia: Churchill Livingstone; 1999. p. 914.
5. Herzberg G, Forissier D. Acute dorsal transscaphoid perilunate fracture-dislocations: medium-term results. J Hand Surg Br 2002;27:498–502.
6. Herzberg G, Comtet JJ, Linscheid RL, et al. Perilunate dislocations and fracture-dislocations: a multicenter study. J Hand Surg Am 1993;18:768–79.
7. Hildebrand KA, Ross DC, Patterson SD, et al. Dorsal perilunate dislocations and fracture-dislocations: questionnaire, clinical, and radiographic evaluation. J Hand Surg Am 2000;25:1069–79.

8. Mayfield JK, Johnson RP, Kilcoyne RK. Carpal dislocations: pathomechanics and progressive perilunar instability. J Hand Surg Am 1980;5:226–41.

9. Najarian R, Nourbakhsh A, Capo JT. Peilunate injuries. Hand (N Y) 2011;6:1–7.

10. Melone CP Jr, Murphy MS, Raskin KB. Perilunate injuries. Repair by dual dorsal and volar approaches. Hand Clin 2000;16:439–48.

11. Herzberg G. Acute dorsal trans-scaphoid perilunate dislocations: open reduction and internal fixation. Tech Hand Up Extrem Surg 2000;4:2–13.

12. Kailu L, Zhou X, Fuguo H. Chronic perilunate dislocations treated with open reduction and internal fixation: results of medium-term follow-up. Int Orthop 2010;34(8):1315–20.

13. Adkison JW, Chapman MW. Treatment of acute lunate and perilunate dislocations. Clin Orthop Relat Res 1982;164:199–207.

14. Apergis E, Maris J, Theodoratos G, et al. Perilunate dislocations and fracture-dislocations. Closed and early open reduction compared in 28 cases. Acta Orthop Scand Suppl 1997;275:55–9.

15. White RE Jr, Omer GE Jr. Transient vascular compromise of the lunate after fracture-dislocation or dislocation of the carpus. J Hand Surg Am 1984;9:181–4.

16. Capo JT, Corti SJ, Tan V. Treatment of dorsal perilunate dislocations and fracture-dislocations using a standardized protocol. Hand (N Y) 2012;7:380–7.

17. Berger RA. A method of defining palpable landmarks for the ligament-splitting dorsal wrist capsulotomy. J Hand Surg 2007;32A:1291–5.

18. Krause DN, Duckles SP, Pelligrino DA. Influence of sex steroid hormones on cerebrovascular function. J Appl Physiol 2006;101:1252–61.

19. Rosenwasser MP, Miyasajsa KC, Strauch RJ. The RASL procedure: reduction and association of the scaphoid and lunate using the Herbert screw. Tech Hand Up Extrem Surg 1997;1:263–72.

20. Souer JS, Rutgers M, Andermahr J, et al. Peilunate fracture-dislocations of the wrist: comparison of temporary screw versus K-wire fixation. J Hand Surg Am 2007;32:318–25.

21. Puttlitz CM, Adams BD, Brown TD. Bioabsorbable pin fixation of intercarpal joints: an evaluation of fixation stiffness. Clin Biomech (Bristol, Avon) 1997;12: 149–53.

22. Forli A, Courvoisier A, Wimsey S, et al. Perilunate dislocations and transscaphoid perilunate fracture-dislocations: a retrospective study with minimum ten-year follow-up. J Hand Surg Am 2010;35:62–8.

23. Nagle DJ. Evaluation of chronic wrist pain. J Am Acad Orthop Surg 2000;8:45–55.

24. Park MJ, Ahn JH. Arthroscopically assisted reduction and percutaneous fixation of dorsal perilunate dislocations and fracture-dislocations. Arthroscopy 2005;21:1153.

Management of Intercarpal Ligament Injuries Associated with Distal Radius Fractures

Mihir J. Desai, MD[a,*], Robin N. Kamal, MD[b],
Marc J. Richard, MD[c,1]

KEYWORDS

- Distal radius fracture • Intercarpal ligament • Scapholunate • Lunotriquetral

KEY POINTS

- There are reports of up to 69% prevalence of intercarpal ligament injury in the setting of distal radius fracture.
- High-grade scapholunate tears impart more long-term symptoms and disability than low-grade tears or lunotriquetral ligament injuries.
- The diagnosis requires a high index of suspicion and begins with radiography and may require advanced imaging such as computed tomography arthrography or MRI. Ultimately, arthroscopy remains the gold standard for diagnosis.
- Optimum management is controversial and should be directed toward ligamentous injuries that create static or dynamic instability or are found on advanced imaging/arthroscopy for clinical suspicion.

INTRODUCTION

Distal radius fractures (DRF) represent 14% of all extremity injuries.[1] These injuries are a common reason for presentation to medical services and are often caused by falling onto an outstretched hand when the wrist is extended, after high-velocity impacts such as those associated with motor vehicle accidents or after minimal trauma in the elderly population.[1–3]

The prevalence of ligamentous injury associated with fractures of the distal radius has been reported to be as high as 69% when partial injuries are included.[4] Injury to the scapholunate interosseous ligament (SLIL) has been reported to occur in 16% to 40% of patients[5–7] and injury to the lunotriquetral interosseous ligament (LTIL) in 8.5% to 15% of patients with distal radius fractures when evaluated arthroscopically.[5,7] Extension into the lunate facet[5] or greater than 2 mm in ulnar positive variance at the time of injury[8] were suggestive of an intercarpal ligament injury.

The SLIL, in conjunction with the LTIL, imparts stability to the proximal row of the carpus. An isolated, complete tear of the SLIL results in scapholunate instability[9–12] and can progress to a predictable pattern of posttraumatic wrist arthritis through a scapholunate advanced collapse pattern.[12] When associated with distal radius

[a] Department of Orthopaedic Surgery, Duke University, 4709 Creekstone Drive, Durham, NC 27703, USA;
[b] Department of Orthopaedic Surgery, Stanford University, 450 Broadway Street Pavilion C, Room c-440, Redwood City, CA 94063, USA; [c] Department of Orthopaedic Surgery, Duke University, 4709 Creekstone Drive, Durham, NC 27703, USA
[1] Senior author.
* Corresponding author. 1215 21st Avenue South, MCE, South Tower Suite, 3200 Nashville, TN 37232.
E-mail address: mihirjdesai@gmail.com

Hand Clin 31 (2015) 409–416
http://dx.doi.org/10.1016/j.hcl.2015.04.009
0749-0712/15/$ – see front matter © 2015 Elsevier Inc. All rights reserved.

fractures, SLIL injury causes progressive deterioration of the intercarpal relationship.[8,13,14]

Multiple reports in the literature describe the types of distal radius fractures associated with intercarpal ligament injuries. Mudgal and Hastings proposed the pathomechanics of combined intercarpal ligamentous injuries and DRF through 2 potential mechanisms.[15] One mechanism is associated with a die-punch fracture and results in compression loading with shear stress across the SLIL. The other mechanism consists of a combination of tensile stress and compression stress at the SLIL resulting from a 4-part distal radius fracture. Mudgal and Jones, using plain radiographs only, described 10 cases of SLIL injury in the setting of 4-part intra-articular distal radius fractures.[16] These authors reported that injuries with die-punch fragments, dorsal comminution, and abnormal scapholunate angle intervals had a high likelihood of SLIL injury. Forward and colleagues[8] reported that grade III SLIL injuries can be associated with ulnar positive variance at the time of initial presentation of a distal radial fracture. These injuries could lead to scapholunate dissociation (SLD) at final follow-up, particularly in patients with intra-articular fractures.

Ogawa and colleagues[17] reported a series in which SLIL and LTIL injuries were present not only in severely comminuted intra-articular fractures but also in minimally displaced extra-articular fractures. Although Mudgal and Hastings[15] only considered intra-articular fractures, similar mechanisms would explain the occurrence of ligamentous injuries in extra-articular fractures.

The utility of standard radiographs in the diagnosis of SLIL injuries has been debated. Kwon and Baek[18] reported that the scapholunate interval was consistently greater in complete SLIL injuries compared with lower-grade injuries and in ulnar deviation compared with radial deviation. They concluded that a scapholunate interval of greater than 2 mm was satisfactory in diagnosing arthroscopy-confirmed Geisler III or IV SLIL injuries.[18] In a survey study of more than 200 surgeons, Gradl and colleagues[19] examined the interobserver reliability, sensitivity, and specificity of radiographs in diagnosing SLIL injuries in the setting of intra-articular distal radius fractures. Each true SLIL injury was confirmed using computed tomography (CT) arthrography or arthroscopy. The authors reported that radiographs are moderately reliable in diagnosing SLIL injuries in distal radius fractures and are better at ruling out these injuries than confirming their presence.[19]

In a comparative study between advanced imaging and radiography, Suzuki and colleagues[20] reported that coronal CT scans were the most effective in diagnosing an arthroscopically confirmed SLIL injury using measurements of the scapholunate interval. They further discussed the limited interobserver reliability of plain radiographs in measuring the scapholunate interval and that the reliability and accuracy improved with the use of CT scans preoperatively.

Some investigators use the standard use of CT arthrography as part of the diagnostic algorithm for patients with intra-articular distal radius fracture and radiographic signs of SLIL.[21,22] Previous studies suggest that CT arthrography of the wrist can detect scapholunate and lunotriquetral ligament injury with a sensitivity of up to 94% and specificity of up to 95%.[19]

High-resolution magnetic resonance imaging (MRI) is now the advanced imaging modality of choice for evaluating the SLIL in most centers.[23] Reliable and accurate MRI diagnosis depends on multiple factors, such as the imaging protocol, the radiologist's experience, and whether the tear is complete or incomplete. MRI, with or without gadolinium injection, is reported to have an average of only 71% sensitivity, 88% specificity, and 84% accuracy in detecting SLIL tears.[24–31] Others have reported a sensitivity of 89% and a specificity of 100% for detecting SL ligament tears using 3 Tesla MRI.[32]

Arthroscopy remains the gold-standard diagnostic tool for determination of intra-articular pathology in the setting of distal radius fractures. SLIL and LTIL injuries are graded by the arthroscopy classification by Geissler (**Table 1**).[5]

Patients with SLIL injury and associated distal radius fractures may have worse wrist function than those with distal radius fracture alone if treated conservatively.[14] Complete SLIL injuries associated with distal radius fractures result in increased scapholunate joint pain and scapholunate dissociation.[8] Early diagnosis of these complete injuries facilitates reduction and repair and may lead to improved outcomes.[33]

SURGICAL TECHNIQUE
Preoperative Planning

The diagnosis of any intercarpal ligament injury begins with a thorough clinical examination. However, the diagnosis of acute ligamentous injury is difficult, especially when associated with a fracture of the distal radius. Fracture-associated pain and concomitant bony instabilities preclude provocative wrist ligament testing.[23] Intercarpal ligament injuries can be diagnosed by various modalities, including radiography, fluoroscopy, arthrography, MRI, and arthroscopy. Although wrist

Table 1
Geissler arthroscopic classification of tears of the intercarpal ligaments

Grade	Description
I	Attenuation or hemorrhage of interosseous ligament—viewed from radiocarpal space No incongruency of carpal alignment in midcarpal space
II	Attenuation of hemorrhage of interosseous ligament—viewed from radiocarpal space Incongruency or step-off of carpal space; slight gap between carpal bones (less than width of probe)
III	Incongruency or step-off of carpal alignment as seen from both radiocarpal and mid-carpal space; probe may be passed between carpal bones
IV	Incongruency or step-off of carpal alignment as seen from both radiocarpal and mid-carpal space; there is gross instability with manipulation; 2.7-mm arthroscope may be passed between carpal bones.

Adapted from Geissler WB, Freeland AE, Savoie FH, et al. Intracarpal soft-tissue lesions associated with an intra-articular fracture of the distal end of the radius. J Bone Joint Surg Am 1996;78:363.

patients with distal radius fractures because of invasiveness and cost. Fluoroscopy may be more appropriate as the initial adjunctive imaging modality because it is noninvasive and inexpensive.

Initially, we obtain high-quality posteroanterior (PA), lateral, and scaphoid radiographs at the time of injury if an intercarpal ligament injury is suspected (**Fig. 1**). Often, contralateral wrist radiographs are necessary for comparison. Radiographic signs of SLD include widening of the scapholunate interval (>2 mm), a scapholunate angle greater than 70°, discontinuity in Gilula's lines, and the presence of a scaphoid ring sign.[35–37] Dynamic imaging, including PA grip views, is typically difficult to obtain with a concomitant distal radius fracture. Imaging should be adequate such that the scapholunate angle and the scapholunate interval can be measured.

If plain radiographs are suggestive of an intercarpal ligament injury, we obtain an MRI preoperatively or perform arthroscopy or dynamic fluoroscopic examination at the time of fracture fixation.[38] Our practice is based on the opinion that in the setting of a concomitant distal radius fracture, the acute management of an SLIL injury with percutaneous or arthroscopically guided Kirschner wire (K-wire) fixation might lead to less pain, disability, and arthrosis.[23,39,40]

Preparation and Patient Positioning

The patient is positioned supine on the operating room table with a hand table under the injured extremity. We use an upper arm tourniquet and standard surgical preparation and draping. If the

arthroscopy is the gold standard for evaluation of the scapholunate and lunotriquetral interval because it can directly evaluate the ligaments and the joint space,[34] it is not performed in all

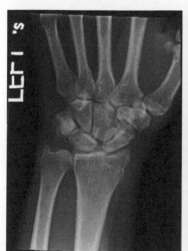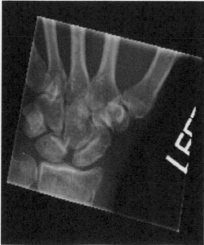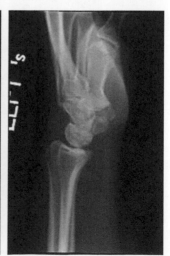

Fig. 1. PA (*left*), oblique (*middle*), and lateral (*right*) wrist radiographs of a polytraumatized patient who was found to have scapholunate widening in the setting of a depressed radial styloid fracture. The diagnosis of SLIL tear was confirmed at the time of surgical treatment.

preoperative imaging is concerning for intercarpal ligament injury, we ensure that wrist arthroscopy equipment is available in the operating room.

Surgical Approach

The surgical approach to these injuries depends primarily on the pattern of the distal radius fracture. We do not routinely perform arthroscopic-assisted reduction unless the fracture pattern involves an isolated, depressed radial styloid fragment. Most commonly, we perform volar plate fixation; however, fragment-specific fixation and dorsal bridge plating are considered for appropriate fracture patterns. For volar plating, we use a standard flexor carpi radialis approach. For bridge plating, we use 3 incisions overlying the (1) proximal radius diaphysis, (2) distal radius metaphysis, and (3) long metacarpal.[41] If the patient has a confirmed intercarpal ligament tear, we use a dorsal incision ulnar to Lister's tubercle or work through the middle incision of the bridge plate to access the injury.

Surgical Procedure

1. Before intraoperative assessment of the intercarpal ligaments, the distal radius fracture is treated with appropriate reduction and fixation.
2. Even if a preoperative MRI shows intercarpal ligament pathology, dynamic stress testing of the carpus is performed to confirm the diagnosis of an intercarpal ligament tear. We obtain PA, lateral, ulnar deviated, and traction views. If

there is any disruption or Gilula's lines or widening of the scapholunate or lunotriquetral interspace, we proceed to surgically address the injury (**Fig. 2**). If the evaluation is equivocal and the surgical procedure does not allow for direct visualization of the injury, arthroscopy is used to evaluate the intercarpal ligaments. Standard radiocarpal and midcarpal arthroscopy are performed.

3. Intercarpal ligament repair—We repair the SLIL using suture anchors in the footprint of the ligament. Before securing the sutures, a large pointed reduction clamp is used to maintain the reduction. The scaphoid typically requires a combination of ulnar translation, extension, and supination to anatomically reduce. After repair, we use K-wire stabilization across the scapholunate interspace. Typically, two 0.045-inch wires are placed percutaneously. For injuries that already have a scaphoid flexion deformity, we add a scaphocapitate pin. Repair of the LTIL is performed in a similar fashion if there is a volar ligament tear. K-wire stabilization is performed across the lunotriquetral articulation. Pins are cut beneath the skin to minimize postoperative complications (**Figs. 3 and 4**).

IMMEDIATE AFTERCARE

The upper extremity is placed in a short arm thumb spica splint for 2 weeks. Digital range of motion is encouraged immediately.

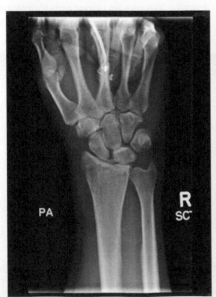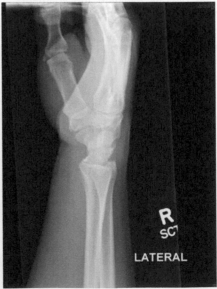

Fig. 2. PA (*left*) and lateral (*right*) wrist radiographs of a distal radius fracture involving the radial styloid and dorsal lunate facet. The lunate facet fracture was a die-punch fracture from direct compression of the lunate into the radius. The scapholunate interval measures 3 mm.

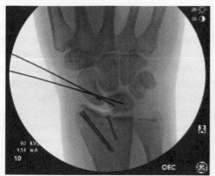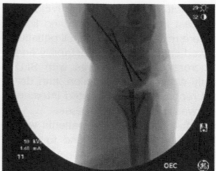

Fig. 3. AP (*left*) and lateral (*right*) intraoperative fluoroscopy images of the same wrist after open reduction and internal fixation of the radial styloid and dorsal lunate facet fracture with Acutrak screws (Acumed, Hillsboro, OR). The lunate facet fracture was approached dorsally, and an SLIL avulsion from the scaphoid was confirmed. The SLIL tear was repaired using a Mitek suture anchor (Raynham, MA). K-wire fixation was used to stabilize the scapholunate articulation.

REHABILITATION AND RECOVERY

Two weeks postoperatively, the patient's sutures are removed, and a short arm thumb spica cast is placed for an additional 4 weeks. At the 6-week mark, the patient is removed from the cast, the pins are removed, and supervised wrist range of motion with an occupational therapist is begun.

CLINICAL RESULTS

The degree to which intercarpal ligament injuries may add to the impairment, symptoms, and disability after recovery from a fracture of the distal radius is debated. Tang and colleagues[14] compared 20 patients with radiographic signs of SLD associated with a DRF with 228 patients with fractures and no signs of intercarpal ligament

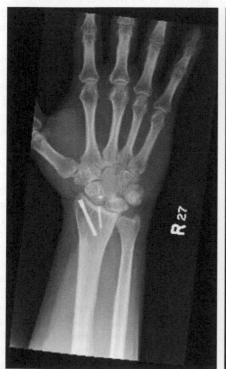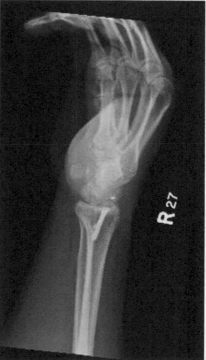

Fig. 4. PA (*left*) and lateral (*right*) of the same wrist 17 months after surgery. The patient reported minimal wrist pain and near symmetric range of motion. Pins were removed 6 weeks postoperatively.

disruption.[14] All fractures were treated with closed reduction and cast immobilization, and no ligament injuries were repaired. At 1 year, all patients with SLD showed signs of chronic instability and significantly increased SLD. Patients with SLD had significantly worse overall function, and delayed ligament reconstruction or limited intercarpal arthrodesis was performed in 8 cases.

In a retrospective review of 839 patients with DRF, 112 (13.4%) patients were found to have persistent SLD after reduction.[42] None of these patients received treatment of their ligamentous injury. At final follow-up, 79 patients had tenderness to palpation over the scapholunate interval with fair to poor outcomes on the Green and O'Brien rating system. The authors concluded that most patients with SLIL injuries and persistent SLD after DRF will be symptomatic. Others have shown that patients with abnormal scapholunate angles at the time of presentation may have signs of static scapholunate dissociation at final follow-up, signifying the high morbidity of these injuries if left untreated.[43]

Advocates of arthroscopically assisted fracture reduction techniques for DRF often cite the ability to acutely diagnose and treat SLIL injuries. In a retrospective review of 26 wrists treated exclusively with arthroscopically assisted fracture fixation using K-wires, the authors also treated 19 SLIL and 10 LTIL injuries.[4] The authors used percutaneous pinning techniques across the intercarpal articulations. They reported an overall 92% satisfaction with this treatment. Of the 19 patients with scapholunate instability managed by K-wire fixation, 9 had a residual diastasis of $\geq$3 mm. There was a significant difference in the incidence of persistent diastasis and the Geissler classification: grade I (0%), II (0%), III (42%), and IV (100%). Others using similar techniques have reported stable scapholunate and lunotriquetral joints after debridement and pinning across the SL and LT articulation when intercarpal ligament tears are diagnosed arthroscopically.[44]

A randomized prospective study compared arthroscopically and fluoroscopically assisted fixation for intra-articular DRF with fluoroscopically assisted fixation alone.[45] Complete or incomplete scapholunate ligament tears were diagnosed and treated in 9 patients in the arthroscopy group. Patients who underwent arthroscopically assisted treatment had significantly better supination, extension, and flexion and a higher mean modified Mayo wrist score at all time points compared with those who had only fluoroscopically treated injuries. The authors concluded that better treatment of associated intra-articular injuries might have been one of the reasons for the improved outcome.

In an effort to define the natural history of intercarpal ligament injuries with DRF, Forward and colleagues[8] conducted a prospective observational study with follow-up of 1 year. The authors performed various forms of DRF fixation including pinning, open reduction and internal fixation, and arthroscopic-assisted reduction. All wrists were examined arthroscopically for the presence of intra-articular injury. The authors reported that an increase of greater than 2 mm in ulnar positive variance at the time of distal radial fracture in a young adult was associated with a 4-fold increase in the risk of scapholunate ligament injury. The study also demonstrated that grade 3 (Geissler III or IV) scapholunate injuries are associated with greater scapholunate joint pain and signs of radiographic dissociation at 1 year after a fracture.

Gradl and colleagues[19] retrospectively compared a cohort of patients with intra-articular DRF and SLIL injury that was diagnosed and treated (N = 18) with a cohort of patients with DRF without associated ligament injury (N = 20).[19] Treatment of the fractures included dorsal plating, volar plating, bridge plating, and closed reduction and percutaneous pinning. SLIL injuries were repaired acutely. The 2 cohorts were compared for differences in motion, grip strength, pain, Mayo wrist score, and Quick Disabilities of the Arm, Shoulder, and Hand score an average of 43 months after surgery. The authors used a radiographic assessment including fracture union, palmar tilt, radial inclination, ulnar variance, intercarpal angles, and the presence of arthrosis. There were no significant differences in the outcome measures between the groups, and the authors concluded that the outcomes of intra-articular DRF with operatively treated associated SLIL injuries are comparable with the outcomes of intra-articular DRF without associated SLIL injuries.

The literature is inconclusive regarding the optimal management of intercarpal injuries in fractures of the distal radius. Some reports support acute treatment, whereas others show fracture treatment alone results in satisfactory outcomes. A potential concern is that if SLIL and LTIL injuries are relatively common, there seems to be limited major sequelae associated with these injuries observed anecdotally in clinical practice. The most obvious explanation is that DRF may impart some residual pain beyond the time to union. This pain may be caused by the fracture or may be owing to injury to the intercarpal ligaments. It is possible that over the years, treatment of DRF included some period of immobilization, which may have adequately treated most carpal ligament injuries. With a trend toward internal fixation of

DRF and early mobilization, these intercarpal ligament injuries may not heal, thereby causing clinical instability and pain.

SUMMARY

The prevalence of ligamentous injury associated with fractures of the distal radius has been reported to be as high as 69% with injury to the SLIL and LTIL reported to occur in 16% to 40% and 8.5% to 15%, respectively. The diagnosis of these injuries begins with standard radiographs but may eventually require advanced imaging such as CT arthrography or MRI based on clinical suspicion. Arthroscopy remains the gold standard diagnostic tool and provides one method for repair of these injuries with fracture fixation. Ultimately, if diagnosed acutely, intercarpal ligament tears can be effectively managed at the time of fracture fixation. Recommendations on the diagnosis and management of intra-articular ligament injuries associated with distal radius fractures are limited. Although those ligament tears that cause static or dynamic instability should be treated with acute repair, the evidence to support the routine use of additional imaging or arthroscopy to diagnose and treat partial tears is limited. Because the outcomes of high-grade (Geissler III/IV) SLIL tears are shown to be poor, a high index of suspicion both preoperatively and postoperatively is required to ensure appropriate treatment of these injuries.

REFERENCES

1. Chen N, Jupiter J. Management of distal radial fractures. J Bone Joint Surg Am 2007;89:2052–62.
2. Trail IA, Stanley JK, Hayton MJ. Twenty questions on carpal instability. J Hand Surg Eur 2007;32(3): 240–55.
3. Hanel DP, Jones MD, Trumble TE. Wrist fractures. Orthop Clin North Am 2002;33(1):35–57.
4. Mehta JA, Bain GI, Heptinstall RJ. Anatomical reduction of intra-articula fractures of the distal radius. An arthroscopically-assisted approach. J Bone Joint Surg Br 2000;82:79–86.
5. Geissler WB, Freeland AE, Savoie FH, et al. Intracarpal soft-tissue lesions associated with an intra-articular fracture of the distal end of the radius. J Bone Joint Surg Am 1996;78:357–65.
6. Peicha G, Seibert F, Fellinger M, et al. Midterm results of arthroscopic treatment of scapholunate ligament lesions associated with intra-articular distal radius fractures. Knee Surg Sports Traumatol Arthrosc 1999;7:327–33.
7. Richards RS, Bennett JD, Roth JH, et al. Arthroscopic diagnosis of intra-articular soft tissue injuries associated with distal radial fractures. J Hand Surg Am 1997;22:772–6.
8. Forward DP, Lindau TR, Melsom DS. Intercarpal ligament injuries associated with fractures of the distal part of the radius. J Bone Joint Surg Am 2007;89: 2334–40.
9. Mitsuyasu H, Patterson RM, Shah MA, et al. The role of the dorsal intercarpal ligament in dynamic and static scapholunate instability. J Hand Surg Am 2004;29:279–88.
10. Short WH, Werner FW, Green JK, et al. Biomechanical evaluation of ligamentous stabilizers of the scaphoid and lunate. J Hand Surg Am 2002;27: 991–1002.
11. Short WH, Werner FW, Green JK, et al. Biomechanical evaluation of the ligamentous stabilizers of the scaphoid and lunate: part II. J Hand Surg Am 2005;30:24–34.
12. Watson HK, Weinzweig J, Zeppieri J. The natural progression of scaphoid instability. Hand Clin 1997;13:39–49.
13. Laulan J, Bismuth JP. Intracarpal ligamentous lesions associated with fractures of the distal radius: outcome at one year: a prospective study of 95 cases. Acta Orthop Belg 1999;65:418–23.
14. Tang JB, Shi D, Gu YQ, et al. Can cast immobilization successfully treat scapholunate dissociation associated with distal radius fractures? J Hand Surg Am 1996;21:583–90.
15. Mudgal C, Hastings H. Scapho-lunate diastasis in fractures of the distal radius. Pathomechanics and treatment options. J Hand Surg Am 1993; 18B:725–9.
16. Mudgal CS, Jones WA. Scapho-lunate diastasis: a component of fractures of the distal radius. J Hand Surg Br 1990;15B:503–5.
17. Ogawa T, Tanaka T, Yanai T, et al. Analysis of soft tissue injuries associated with distal radius fractures. BMC Sports Sci Med Rehabil 2013;5:19–22.
18. Kwon BC, Baek GH. Fluoroscopic Diagnosis of Scapholunate Inerosseous Ligament Injuries in Distal Radius Fractures. Clin Orthop Relat Res 2008;466: 969–76.
19. Gradl G, Neuhaus V, Fuchsberge T, et al. Radiographic diagnosis of scapholunate dissociation among intra-articular fractures of the distal radius: interobserver reliability. J Hand Surg Am 2013;38A: 1685–90.
20. Suzuki D, Ono H, Furuta K, et al. Comparison of scapholunate distance measurements on plain radiography and computed tomograpghy for the diagnosis of scapholunate instability associated with distal radius fracture. J Orthop Sci 2014;19: 465–70.
21. Theumann N, Favarger N, Schnyder P, et al. Wrist ligament injuries: value of post-arthrography computed tomography. Skeletal Radiol 2001;30:88–93.

22. Bille B, Harley B, Cohen H. A comparison of CT arthrography of the wrist to findings during wrist arthroscopy. J Hand Surg Am 2007;32A:834–41.

23. Kitay A, Wolfe SW. Scapholunate instability: current concepts in diagnosis and management. J Hand Surg Am 2012;37:2175–96.

24. Schmid MR, Scherter T, Pfirrmann CW, et al. Interosseous ligament tears of the wrist: comparison of multi-detector row CT arthrograpghy and MR imaging. Radiology 2005;237:1008–13.

25. Smith DK. Volar carpal ligaments of the wrist: normal appearance on multiplanar reconstructions of three-dimensional Fourier transform MR imaging. AJR Am J Roentgenol 1993;161:353–7.

26. Berger RA, Linscheid RL, Berquist TH. Magnetic resonance imaging of the anterior radiocarpal ligaments. J Hand Surg 1994;19A:295–303.

27. Scheck RJ, Kubitzek C, Hierner R, et al. The scapholunate interosseous ligament in MR arthrography of the wrist: correlation with non-enhanced MRI and wrist arthroscopy. Skeletal Radiol 1997;26:263–71.

28. Zanetti M, Saupe N, Nagy L. Role of MR imaging in chronic wrist pain. Eur Radiol 2007;17:927–38.

29. Schadel-Hopfner M, Iwinska-Zelder J, Braus T, et al. MRI versus arthroscopy in the diagnosis of scapholunate ligament injury. J Hand Surg 2001;26B:17–21.

30. Haims AH, Schweitzer ME, Morrison WB, et al. Internal derangement of the wrist: indirect MR arthrography versus unenhanced MR imaging. Radiology 2003;227:701–7.

31. Manton GL, Schweitzer ME, Weishaupt D, et al. Partial interosseous ligament tears of the wrist: difficulty in utilizing either primary or secondary MRI signs. J Comput Assist Tomogr 2001;25:671–6.

32. Magee T. Comparison of 3-T MRI and arthroscopy of intrinsic wrist ligament and TFCC tears. AJR Am J Roentgenol 2009;192:80–5.

33. Whipple TL. The role of arthroscopy in the treatment of scapholunate instability. Hand Clin 1995; 11:37–40.

34. Garcia-Elias M, An KN, Amadio PC, et al. Reliability of carpal angle determinations. J Hand Surg Am 1989;14:1017–21.

35. Schimmerl-Metz SM, Metz VM, Totterman SM, et al. Radiologic measurement of the scapholunate joint: implications of biologic variation in scapholunate joint morphology. J Hand Surg Am 1999;24(6): 1237–44.

36. Pliefke J, Stengel D, Rademacher G, et al. Diagnostic accuracy of plain radiographs and cineradiography in diagnosing traumatic scapholunate dissociation. Skeletal Radiol 2008;37(2):139–45.

37. Megerle K, Pohlmann S, Kloeters O, et al. The significance of conventional radiographic parameters in the diagnosis of scapholunate ligament lesions. Eur Radiol 2011;21(1):176–81.

38. Kwon BC, Choi SJ, Song SY, et al. Modified carpal stretch test as a screening test for detection of scapholunate interosseous ligament injuries associated with distal radius fractures. J Bone Joint Surg Am 2011;93:855–62.

39. Walsh JJ, Berger RA, Cooney WP. Current status of scapholunate interosseous ligament injuries. J Am Acad Orthop Surg 2002;10:32–42.

40. Darlis NA, Kaufmann RA, Giannoulis F, et al. Arthroscopic debridement and closed pinning for chronic dynamic scapholunate instability. J Hand Surg 2006; 31A:418–24.

41. Ruch DS, Ginn TA, Yang CC, et al. Use of a distraction plate for distal radial fractures with metaphyseal and diaphyseal comminution. J Bone Joint Surg Am 2005;87:945–54.

42. Gunal I, Ozaksoy D, Altay T, et al. Scapholunate dissociation associated with distal radius fractures. Eur J Orthop Surg Traumatol 2013;23:877–81.

43. Bunker DL, Pappas G, Moradi P, et al. Radiographic signs of static carpal instability with distal end radius fractures: is current treatment adequate? Hand Surg 2012;17:325–30.

44. Shih JT, Lee HM, Hou YT, et al. Arthroscopically-assisted reduction of intra-articular fractures and soft tissue management of distal radius. Hand Surg 2001;6:127–35.

45. Varitimidis SE, Basdekis GK, Dailiana ZH, et al. Treatment of intra-articular fractures of the distal radius: fluoroscopic or arthroscopic reduction? J Bone Joint Surg Br 2008;90:778–85.

Acute Scapholunate Ligament Injuries
Arthroscopic Treatment

John M. Bednar, MD*

KEYWORDS

- Scapholunate ligament • Wrist arthroscopy • Carpal instability • Scapholunate instability

KEY POINTS

- Anatomically, the scapholunate interosseous ligament (SLIL) has 3 distinct regions, each with a different histologic appearance and different biomechanical properties; the dorsal component of the SLIL has the highest strength to failure.
- Wrist arthroscopy allows assessment of all 3 components of the SLIL with greater accuracy than can be obtained through radiographic or MRI evaluation.
- Partial acute injuries to the SLIL are treated arthroscopically with debridement and electrothermal shrinkage with a high degree of success and patient satisfaction.
- A complete tear of the SLIL can be treated with arthroscopic reduction and fixation with a high degree of success if treated within 3 months of injury.

 Videos of arthroscopic views of the proximal scapholunate (SL) ligament and dorsal SL ligament; arthroscopic examinations of Geissler SLIL injuries; arthroscopic debridement of a proximal SLIL tear; arthroscopic reduction of SL interval; arthroscopic view of second SL K-wire; and fluoroscopy video of K-wire placement across SL interval accompany this article at http://www.hand.theclinics.com/

INTRODUCTION

The early diagnosis and treatment of acute scapholunate (SL) ligament injuries continues to be a challenge. Berger[1] defined the anatomy of the SL interosseous ligament (SLIL). He described the ligament having 3 distinct regions. The central (proximal) membranous portion (**Fig. 1**, Video 1; available online at http://www.hand.theclinics.com/) is cartilaginous with a few longitudinal fibers. The dorsal portion of the interosseous ligament (**Fig. 2**, Video 2; available online at http://www.hand.theclinics.com/) is histologically a true ligament. It is composed of stout transverse fibers

and is the thickest portion of the SLIL. The palmar (volar) portion of the interosseous ligament (**Fig. 3**) is also histologically a true ligament, 1 to 2 mm thick, and composed of longer oblique fibers that allow rotation in the sagittal plane.

Biomechanically the dorsal SLIL has the highest strength to failure. It is the most important portion of the SLIL for constraining rotation, translation, and distraction between the scaphoid and lunate. The palmar segment is an important constraint to rotation of the SL joint. The proximal portion provides no significant constraint to the SL joint.

However, the stability of the SL joint is not provided by just the SLIL but depends on a complex

Conflicts of Interest: The author has no conflicts to disclose.
Department of Orthopaedic Surgery, The Philadelphia Hand Center (South Jersey Hand Center), Thomas Jefferson University Hospital, 1888 Marlton Pike East, Cherry Hill, NJ 08003, USA
* The Philadelphia Hand Center (South Jersey Hand Center), 1888 Marlton Pike East, Cherry Hill, NJ 08003.
E-mail address: jmbednar@handcenters.com

Hand Clin 31 (2015) 417–423
http://dx.doi.org/10.1016/j.hcl.2015.04.001
0749-0712/15/$ – see front matter © 2015 Elsevier Inc. All rights reserved.

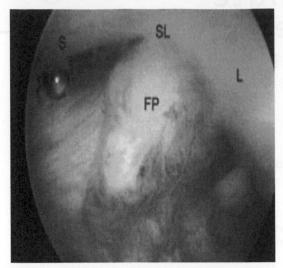

Fig. 1. Arthroscopic view of scaphoid (S), lunate (L), Scapholunate (SL) proximal ligament, and fat pad (FP).

of ligaments, each having a separate role but working together to support the carpus in proper alignment. Short and colleagues[2] determined that the SLIL is the primary stabilizer of the SL articulation and that the dorsal radiocarpal ligament, dorsal intercarpal ligament, scaphotrapezial ligaments, and radioscaphocapitate ligaments are secondary stabilizers.

Mayfield[3] showed that the SLIL can stretch up to 225% its length before eventually tearing. An isolated injury to the SLIL initially may not cause disassociation and widening on plain or stress radiographs. A combined injury to both the intrinsic and extrinsic ligaments will cause a SL diastasis. In patients with isolated SLIL injuries, plain radiograph abnormalities may not be seen initially but

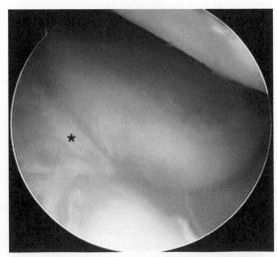

Fig. 2. Arthroscopic view of dorsal SLIL (*asterisk*).

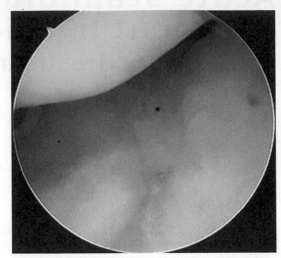

Fig. 3. Arthroscopic view of volar (palmar) SLIL (*asterisk*).

will occur over time as gradual attenuation of the extrinsic ligaments occurs.

Geissler and colleagues[4] proposed an arthroscopic grading scale to quantify the spectrum of instability resulting from injury to carpal interosseous ligaments. This classification is applicable for SLIL injuries.

Geissler arthroscopic classification of carpal instability:

- Grade I: a 1-mm hook probe can be inserted between the scaphoid and lunate (Video 3; available online at http://www.hand.theclinics.com/)
- Grade II: the probe can be rotated 90° from ligament attenuation but a tear may not be visualized (Video 4; available online at http://www.hand.theclinics.com/)
- Grade III: abnormal scaphoid flexion and lunate extension produces a midcarpal step-off at the SL joint when viewed through the midcarpal ulnar (MCU) portal (Video 5; available online at http://www.hand.theclinics.com/)
- Grade IV: a complete SLIL tear allows the arthroscope to pass from the radiocarpal to the midcarpal joint when the scope is in the 3–4 portal (Video 6; available online at http://www.hand.theclinics.com/)

Management based on the Geissler arthroscopic classification:

- Grade I: immobilization/thermal shrinkage
- Grade II: debridement/thermal shrinkage arthroscopic reduction and fixation
- Grade III: arthroscopic/open reduction fixation and repair

- Grade IV: open reduction and repair tendon graft reconstruction

SURGICAL TECHNIQUE

Standard wrist arthroscopy is performed with the patient supine and the affected extremity placed into a wrist traction apparatus. A complete diagnostic arthroscopy is performed evaluating the radiocarpal and midcarpal joints to identify any coexistent lesions. The membranous central (proximal) portion of the SLIL ligament is best visualized when the arthroscope is placed in the 3–4 radiocarpal portal. The dorsal SLIL is best visualized with the scope in the MCU portal, allowing a probe to be placed through the midcarpal radial (MCR) portal to assess ligament tension. The volar SLIL is evaluated with the scope in the MCR portal.

COMMON SCAPHOLUNATE INTEROSSEOUS LIGAMENT INJURY PATTERNS AND ARTHROSCOPIC TREATMENT
Tear of the Proximal Scapholunate Interosseous Ligament

The tear is debrided using a shaver in the 3–4 radiocarpal portal with the scope in the 4–5 portal (**Fig. 4**, Video 7; available online at http://www.hand.theclinics.com/). After debridement of the frayed ligament the remaining portion may need to be tightened using radiofrequency electrothermal shrinkage. When performing thermal shrinkage, adequate fluid flow must be maintained to prevent heat-generated collagen necrosis and chondrolysis.

Partial Tear of the Dorsal Scapholunate Interosseous Ligament

The tear is debrided with the shaver in the MCR portal with the scope in the MCU portal. After debridement the stability of the SL joint is assessed using the Geissler classification. Geissler type II injuries are treated with arthroscopic reduction of SL alignment and fixation. The lax dorsal SLIL is tightened with thermal shrinkage using a bipolar radiofrequency probe placed through the MCR portal (**Fig. 5**).

Partial Tear of the Volar Scapholunate Interosseous Ligament

The tear is visualized with the scope in either the MCR portal or the volar radial portal.

When using dorsal portals, the scope is placed in the MCU portal and the shaver or radiofrequency probe in the MCR portal. Visualization of the volar ligament can be obstructed by a type 2 lunate requiring the use of a volar portal.

When the volar portal is used for the scope, the shaver or radiofrequency probe is placed through the MCR portal.

Complete Tear of the Dorsal Scapholunate Interosseous Ligament

The dorsal SLIL tear and SL malalignment are visualized with the scope in the MCU portal. The SLIL rupture produces a step-off at the midcarpal SL joint because of scaphoid flexion and rotation (**Fig. 6**). The ligament is debrided. The scaphoid is reduced to the lunate (**Fig. 7**, Video 8; available online at http://www.hand.theclinics.com/) either by external pressure on the scaphoid or using K-wire joysticks placed into the scaphoid and lunate. A 2-cm longitudinal incision is made in the anatomic snuffbox over the scaphoid. Blunt dissection is made to the joint capsule identifying and retracting the radial sensory nerve and radial artery. Two 1.57-mm (0.062-inch) K-wires are

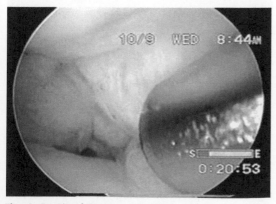

Fig. 4. Proximal SL tear debrided with the shaver in the MCR portal with the scope in the MCU portal.

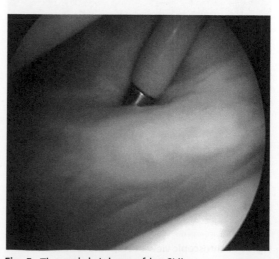

Fig. 5. Thermal shrinkage of lax SLIL.

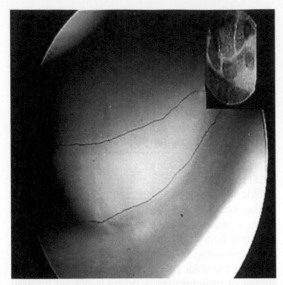

Fig. 6. Arthroscopic view of step-off at the midcarpal SL joint caused by scaphoid flexion and rotation.

placed under fluoroscopic guidance into the scaphoid (**Fig. 8**, Videos 9 and 10; available online at http://www.hand.theclinics.com/) aligned to allow passage across the SL interval into the lunate. The wires are passed into the lunate, closing the SL gap and restoring proper scaphoid rotation and SL alignment (**Figs. 9** and **10**). The arthroscope in the MCU portal allows visualization of the reduction and alignment as the wires are passed into the lunate. The K-wires are bent and either buried under the skin or left exposed.

An alternative technique is to secure the SL interval with a cannulated headless screw (**Fig. 11**).

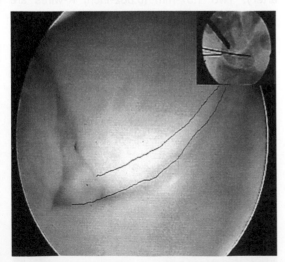

Fig. 7. Arthroscopic view of scaphoid reduction to the lunate.

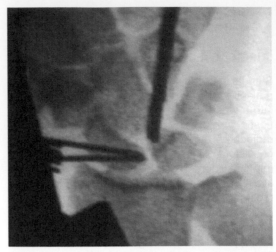

Fig. 8. Fluoroscopy view of two 1.57-mm (0.062-inch) K-wires in the scaphoid aligned to allow fixation of the lunate.

A guidewire for a cannulated headless screw is used as one of the reduction wires with placement of a headless screw across the SL interval allowing removal of the K-wires.

Complete Tear of the Scapholunate Interosseous Ligament

Corella and colleagues[5] described an arthroscopic ligamentoplasty of the dorsal and volar portions of the SL ligament for Geissler III and IV injuries. The technique uses a distally based flexor carpi radialis

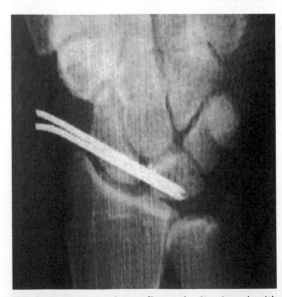

Fig. 9. Anteroposterior radiograph. SL pinned with scaphoid position corrected to close the SL gap and restore scaphoid extension.

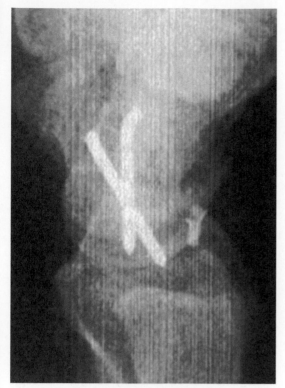

Fig. 10. Lateral radiograph showing normal SL angle with proper alignment of the proximal row.

(FCR) tendon graft. Under arthroscopic guidance a 1-mm K-wire is placed through the 3–4 portal to create the scaphoid tunnel. The K-wire enters the dorsal portion of the scaphoid at the insertion point for the dorsal SLIL. The exit point for the K-wire is

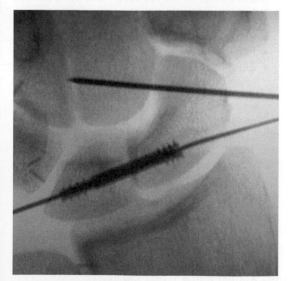

Fig. 11. Fluoroscopy view of cannulated screw placement to secure the SL interval.

the volar scaphoid tuberosity. A 3-mm cannulated drill is run over the K-wire to create the scaphoid tunnel. The lunate tunnel is also created with a 3-mm cannulated drill. The tunnel runs from the dorsal medial region of the lunate in a volar direction parallel to the articular surface of the SL joint. A distally based hemitendon graft, 3 mm wide by 8 to 10 cm long, is harvested from the FCR, being careful to dissect the graft distal to the scaphoid tunnel. A suture lasso entering the 3–4 portal placed through the scaphoid tunnel retrieves the FCR graft, pulling it through the scaphoid. Tension on the graft corrects scaphoid flexion. A biotenodesis screw is placed at the volar exit of the scaphoid tunnel to set the FCR tension. The graft is then captured by a loop that connects the dorsal lunate tunnel with the 3–4 portal passing the graft to the dorsal entrance of the lunate tunnel. A volar skin incision is made over the volar wrist centered over the radial side of the ring metacarpal. Dissection to the volar wrist capsule passes through the flexor tendons retracting the ring and small flexor tendons in an ulnar direction. A volar wrist capsule portal is then made centered over the volar lunate portal. A suture lasso passes the FCR graft through the lunate from dorsal to volar. Under arthroscopic vision the graft is tensioned to close the SL interval and a biotenodesis screw is placed in the dorsal lunate tunnel. A volar capsuloligamentous suture attaches the graft to the volar capsule at the graft's exit from the volar lunate tunnel. The graft is then passed to the volar radial carpal joint proximal to the capsuloligamentous suture. The graft is tensioned to close the volar SL gap and is sutured to adjacent capsuloligamentous tissue.

REHABILITATION AND RECOVERY

Patients treated with debridement and thermal shrinkage are immobilized after surgery in a short-arm thumb spica cast or splint for 2 to 3 weeks. Protected-motion therapy is performed from 3 to 6 weeks after surgery. At 6 weeks all immobilization is stopped and resistive strengthening exercise and functional therapy instituted.

Patients treated with arthroscopic reduction and pinning are immobilized in a short-arm thumb spica cast for 6 to 8 weeks until the K-wires are removed. After K-wire removal, a removable wrist splint is used as therapy progresses to improve wrist motion and strength. Return to sports and heavy use can be anticipated at 3 to 4 months after surgery.

Patients treated with arthroscopic reduction and cannulated screw stabilization of the SL interval are immobilized for 2 to 3 weeks after surgery in a short-arm thumb spica cast. After cast removal, a removable wrist splint is used as wrist motion exercise begins for the next 3 weeks. All splinting can be stopped at 6 weeks as resistive exercise is instituted. Return to regular activities is anticipated at 3 to 4 months after surgery.

The published protocol[5] for the arthroscopic ligamentoplasty recommends immobilization of the wrist for 2 weeks with immediate finger motion exercise. At 2 weeks the patient begins the dart thrower's motion exercise for the wrist and is immobilized in a thermoplastic splint. At 4 weeks, a therapy program involving complete range of wrist motion is started. At 6 weeks, the splint is removed and the patient begins strengthening exercise. Resistance exercises begin at 10 weeks, and normal activities (except contact sports) begin at 12 weeks after surgery. Contact sports are allowed after the fourth or fifth month after surgery.

CLINICAL RESULTS IN THE LITERATURE
Arthroscopic Debridement

At mean follow-up of 27 months, Weiss and colleagues[6] reported satisfactory improvement (symptoms resolved or only occasional symptoms with heavy use) in:

- Eleven of 13 patients (85%) treated by arthroscopic debridement of partial SLIL tear
- Ten of 15 (67%) patients treated with debridement of a complete tear

At a minimum 2 year follow-up, Ruch and Poehling[7] reported satisfactory improvement in:

- All 7 patients treated with arthroscopic debridement of a partial SLIL tear
- No progression to instability seen at final follow-up

Arthroscopic Debridement and Thermal Shrinkage

Darlis and colleagues[8] reported the results of 16 patients with Geissler I and II SL injuries treated by debridement and thermal shrinkage using a bipolar radiofrequency probe.

- Fourteen patients had a partial tear of the membranous (proximal) or volar part of the ligament
- Two patients had a redundant ligament

At a mean follow-up of 19 months:

- Eight patients had complete pain relief
- Fourteen patients reported substantial improvement
- Two patients reported no change in pain
- Mean flexion extension arc was 142°

- Mean grip strength was 78% of the unaffected side
- No radiographic signs of arthritis or static instability were seen at final follow-up

Lee and colleagues[9] reported the results of a retrospective study of 16 wrists in 14 patients with 3 Geissler I and 13 Geissler II SL injuries treated with arthroscopic debridement and thermal shrinkage:

- Mean follow-up was 52.8 months
- Pain visual analog scales were significantly improved from preoperative levels
- Mean flexion extension arc was 136.5°
- Mean postoperative grip strength was 48 kg (106 pounds), which was significantly improved from preoperative levels
- Mayo wrist score improved from 70 before surgery to 94.7 after surgery
- No patient had radiographic evidence of arthritis or instability

Arthroscopic Reduction and Fixation

Whipple[10] reported the results of arthroscopic management of SL instability using arthroscopic reduction and multiple K-wire pinning. Forty patients followed for 1 to 3 years were divided into 2 distinct groups according to duration of symptoms and the SL gap seen on radiographs:

- Group 1: SL instability for less than 3 months, and a 3mm or less gap in SL interval
- Group 2: SL instability for greater than 3 months, or a greater than 3 mm SL gap

Maintenance of the reduction and symptomatic relief:

- Eighty-three percent of group 1 patients
- Fifty-three percent of group 2 patients
- Eighty-five percent of group 1 patients followed for 2 to 7 years continued to maintain their stability in this series

This report emphasized the need for early diagnosis and management for acute SL instability, and the diminished capacity for healing after the injury becomes chronic.

Arthroscopic Ligamentoplasty

Corella and colleagues[5] reported on an arthroscopic technique for the reconstruction of both the dorsal and volar segments of the SLIL. Their report includes an illustrative case of a 37-year-old woman with a 1-year-old injury:

- No loss of preoperative wrist motion

- Visual analog pain score improved from 8 to 1.2
- Disabilities of the Arm, Shoulder, and Hand score improved from 51.8 to 10

A large study with long-term follow-up is needed to assess this technique.

SUMMARY

Wrist arthroscopy is a valuable adjunct to the management of wrist disorders. It enables the evaluation of intracarpal structures with minimal morbidity compared with an arthrotomy. It is an extremely sensitive technique for detecting the spectrum of injury that occurs to the SLIL as it stretches and eventually tears.

Acute partial injuries to the SLIL are treated with debridement and thermal shrinkage with a high percentage of successful results.

Complete SLIL injuries are more significant and more difficult to treat. Acute injuries can be successfully treated by arthroscopic reduction and fixation if treated within 3 months of injury.

Arthroscopic-assisted SLIL reconstruction of the dorsal and volar components of the SLIL using the FCR tendon has been described with encouraging early results. A larger study with long-term follow-up is needed to confirm the value of this technique for treating this difficult clinical problem.

SUPPLEMENTARY DATA

Supplementary data related to this article can be found online at http://dx.doi.org/10.1016/j.hcl.2015.04.001.

REFERENCES

1. Berger RA. The gross and histologic anatomy of the scapholunate interosseous ligament. J Hand Surg Am 1996;21(2):170–8.
2. Short WH, Werner FW, Green JK, et al. Biomechanical evaluation of the ligamentous stabilizers of the scaphoid and lunate: part III. J Hand Surg Am 2007;32:297–309.
3. Mayfield JK. Wrist ligamentous anatomy and pathogenesis of carpal instability. Orthop Clin North Am 1984;15(2):209–16.
4. Geissler WB, Freeland AE, Savoie FH, et al. Intracarpal soft-tissue lesions associated with intra-articular distal radial fractures. J Bone Joint Surg Am 1996;78(3):357–65.
5. Corella F, Del Cerro M, Ocampos M, et al. Arthroscopic ligamentoplasty of the dorsal and volar portions of the scapholunate ligament. J Hand Surg Am 2013;38(12):2466–77.
6. Weiss AP, Sachar K, Glowacki KA. Arthroscopic management of partial scapholunate and lunotriquetral injuries of the wrist. J Hand Surg Am 1997;22:344–9.
7. Ruch DS, Poehling GG. Arthroscopic management of partial scapholunate and lunotriquetral injuries of the wrist. J Hand Surg Am 1996;21:412–7.
8. Darlis NA, Weisser RW, Sotereanos DG. Partial scapholunate ligament injuries treated with arthroscopic debridement and thermal shrinkage. J Hand Surg Am 2005;30(5):908–14.
9. Lee JL, Nha KW, Lee GY, et al. Long-term outcomes of arthroscopic debridement and thermal shrinkage for isolated partial intercarpal ligament tears. Orthopedics 2012;35(8):1204–9.
10. Whipple TL. The role of arthroscopy in the treatment of scapholunate instability. Hand Clin 1995;11(1):37–40.

Open Treatment of Acute Scapholunate Instability

Morgan M. Swanstrom, MD, Steve K. Lee, MD*

KEYWORDS

- Scapholunate • Carpal instability • Wrist

KEY POINTS

- Treatment of scapholunate instability in the acute phase is integral to prevent dorsal intercalated segment instability and advanced degenerative changes.
- In the acute setting, with adequate ligament present, direct scapholunate ligament repair combined with a "double-dorsal" capsulodesis is the favored treatment option for scapholunate instability.
- Literature review reveals that direct scapholunate ligament repair in acute cases of scapholunate instability can produce reasonable clinical outcomes.

INTRODUCTION

Nature of the Problem

Carpal instability is a condition that can lead to significant dysfunction and pain if not treated appropriately. Injury to the scapholunate (SL) ligament complex can lead to dorsal intercalated segment instability and SL advanced collapse (SLAC). For this reason, it is important to understand this joint in context with its contribution to carpal mechanics as well as understand the importance of accurate diagnosis to lead to appropriate and timely treatment.

Relevant Anatomy

The carpus is a complex collection of 8 bones and the anatomic interaction of these articulations produces normal wrist motion and function. The scaphoid and lunate function in this integrated unit to provide motion between carpal segments.[1–3] With regard to the row concept of carpal movement, the scaphoid and lunate belong to the proximal row, and the scaphoid also acts as an intermediary stabilizer of the midcarpal joint between the proximal row and distal row.[4–6] These anatomic relationships are integral to the delicate balance of the wrist with a combination of osseous anatomy and important stabilizing ligamentous structures.[7]

The SL articulation involves a combination of primary and secondary stabilizers. The primary stabilizer of the SL joint is the SL interosseous ligament (SLIL),[8,9] with the biggest strength contribution coming from the dorsal SL ligament[9] followed by the palmar SL ligament and followed then by the proximal membrane. Secondary stabilizers include the radioscaphocapitate, long and short radiolunate, scaphocapitate, radioscapholunate, ulnolunate, ulnotriquetral, scaphotrapeziotrapezoid, dorsal radiotriquetral, and dorsal intercarpal ligaments.[3,4,8,10–13]

Evaluation of Acute Injury

The common mechanism of acute SL injury is a fall onto a wrist positioned in extension, ulnar deviation, and carpal supination. Classifying an injury as acute typically involves a time interval from injury to diagnosis of 6 weeks or less. In the acute setting, there is swelling around the dorsoradial wrist along with tenderness to palpation over the dorsal SL interval and possibly the anatomic snuffbox. A patient with SL pathology usually has pain with wrist loading in the extended position (pushup-type maneuver) and may report a

Hospital for Special Surgery, Hand and Upper Extremity Service, 523 East 72nd Street, New York, NY 10021, USA
* Corresponding author.
E-mail address: steve.kichul.lee@gmail.com

Hand Clin 31 (2015) 425–436
http://dx.doi.org/10.1016/j.hcl.2015.04.008
0749-0712/15/$ – see front matter © 2015 Elsevier Inc. All rights reserved.

sensation of weakness.[14] The scaphoid shift test is useful for clinical diagnosis,[14,15] as is the SL ballottement test.[3] In the scaphoid shift test, the examiner places pressure on the palmar tuberosity of the scaphoid while taking the wrist from ulnar deviation to radial deviation. In a positive test, there is a palpable sensation of the scaphoid subluxating dorsally out of the scaphoid fossa of the radius and when pressure is removed, the scaphoid reduces back. The contralateral side should be tested also; asymmetrical laxity is necessary for a positive test. This maneuver should also reproduce pain in the SL region.[3,16] It is important to acknowledge, though, that in the acute setting, pain may limit provocative examination maneuvers.

With SL dissociation, there are 4 planes of instability: coronal (SL gap), sagittal (scaphoid flexion and lunate extension: dorsal intercalated segment instability [DISI]), translational (dorsal translation of the scaphoid; possibly riding on top of the dorsal ridge of the scaphoid fossa, which is best seen on sagittal advanced imaging of MRI or computed tomography [CT]), and rotational (scaphoid pronation). The most obvious signs radiographically are of the coronal plane instability with asymmetric SL interval widening and of the sagittal plane instability with a flexed scaphoid and an asymmetrically increased SL angle on the lateral view,[3,4,17,18] as well as a scaphoid "ring sign" on the posterior-anterior (PA) view. The best dynamic radiographic view and arguably the best view for overall SL pathology on radiographs is the bilateral clenched pencil view.[19,20] In addition to dynamically loading the SL joint (by ulnarly deviating and driving the capitate between the scaphoid and lunate via joint reaction force), the clenched pencil view also gives a bilateral wrist view and slightly pronates the wrists out of supination to give a true PA view showing the facets of the SL joints. The authors' preferred radiographic views are PA, lateral, oblique, bilateral clench pencil view, and scaphoid view.

When the diagnosis is in question, high-resolution MRI with a 3-T magnet and dedicated wrist coil produces acceptable sensitivity and specificity for diagnosis of SL injury.[21–25] Lower-resolution MRI scans, however, often do not provide enough information to diagnose carpal ligament lesions.[26–28] Depending on the surgeon's preference, diagnostic arthroscopy also can be used if the diagnosis remains in question.

Natural History

Loss of competency of the secondary scaphoid stabilizers, either acutely or via attenuation over time, typically leads to DISI.[29] In this process, the lunate and triquetrum abnormally extend (with radial deviation and supination) while the scaphoid rotates into palmarflexion with its proximal pole subluxated dorsoradially out of the scaphoid fossa of the distal radius. These dissociative changes cause derangements in force transmission across the wrist which then cause SLAC, a degenerative process leading to characteristic patterns of cartilage wear and arthritis.[30] These late-stage changes may require salvage procedures (**Table 1**); thus, it is best to diagnose SL injury in the acute setting to allow for early treatment and decrease the progression of SLAC arthritis.

SURGICAL TECHNIQUE
Preoperative Planning

Preoperative planning involves a history and mechanism of injury, as well as determination of whether the injury is acute ($\leq$6 weeks from injury) or chronic. Physical examination and diagnostic imaging is performed as previously discussed. If the injury is acute, there should be a satisfactory ligament for repair. Requirements for repair include a robust repairable ligament, a reducible carpus, and the absence of degenerative changes.[31]

Preparation and Patient Positioning

Standard patient positioning is supine with a hand table. Regional anesthesia is typically used in combination with conscious sedation. A nonsterile upper-arm tourniquet is applied. Standard preparation is used for the surgical site, and preoperative antibiotic prophylaxis is given in concordance with the patient's allergy profile. Mini-C arm fluoroscopy is draped in a sterile fashion for the procedure.

Surgical Approach

The upper extremity is first exsanguinated with an Esmarch bandage. A dorsal approach to wrist is performed. A 6-cm to 7-cm longitudinal skin incision is made dorsally in line with the third ray centered on the radiocarpal joint. The extensor retinaculum is then exposed, the extensor pollicis longus is released from the third dorsal compartment and retracted radially. The second and fourth dorsal compartments are mobilized radially and ulnarly, respectively. A surgical tip for better exposure of the radial side of the wrist is to mobilize the extensor carpi radialis brevis (ECRB) tendon separately from the extensor carpi radialis longus (ECRL) tendon. Retract the ECRB tendon ulnarly and the ECRL tendon radially for radial-sided wrist exposure and retract both ECRB and ECRL tendons radially for ulnar-sided wrist exposure.

Table 1
Patterns and treatment of SL instability

Patterns and Treatment of Scapholunate Instability	Stage				
	I. Occult	II. Dynamic	III. Scapholunate Dissociation	IV. DISI	V. SLAC
Injured ligaments	Partial SLIL	Incompetent or complete SLIL; partial volar extrinsics	Complete SLIL, volar or dorsal extrinsics	Complete SLIL volar extrinsics; secondary changes in RL, ST, DIC ligaments	As in stage IV
Radiographs	Normal	Usually normal	SL gap ≥3 mm; RS angle ≥60°	SL angle ≥70° SL gap ≥3 mm RL ≥15° CL ≥15°	I. Styloid DJD II. RS DJD III. CL DJD IV. Pancarpal DJD
Stress radiographs	Normal: abnormal fluoroscopy	Abnormal	Grossly abnormal	Unnecessary	Unnecessary
Treatment	Pinning or capsulodesis	SLIL repair with capsulodesis	SLIL repair with capsulodesis vs triligament reconstruction	Reducible: triligament reconstruction Fixed: intercarpal fusion	Intercarpal fusion or proximal row carpectomy

Abbreviations: CL, capitolunate; DIC, dorsal intercarpal ligament; DISI, dorsal intercalated segment instability; DJD, degenerative joint disease; RL, radiolunate; RS, radioscaphoid; SL, scapholunate; SLAC, SL advanced collapse; SLIL, SL interosseous ligament; ST, scaphotrapezoid.
From Kitay A, Wolfe SW. Scapholunate instability: current concepts in diagnosis and management. J Hand Surg Am 2012;37(10):2184; with permission.

Posterior interosseous neurectomy is performed, resecting a 2-cm segment of the nerve at the radial floor of the fourth compartment.

Deep exposure of the carpus is performed using a modification of the Szabo dorsal intercarpal ligament (DIC) technique.[32] We use an ulnar-based capsulotomy flap, raising the capsule from the dorsal rim of the radius proximally and from the distal border of the DIC distally. The radial limb is at the radial border of the carpus (careful hemostasis with bipolar cautery is required here). The capsular flap is carefully dissected off of the insertions on the carpal bones, taking care not to injure the carpal ligaments. This flap is then bisected, dividing it into 2 limbs to be used as a "double-dorsal capsulodesis." The distal limb will be attached to the distal pole of the scaphoid as in the Szabo DIC capsulodesis and the proximal limb will be used as reinforcing capsulodesis for the dorsal SL joint after SL ligament repair is performed (**Figs. 1** and **2**).

Intraoperative evaluation of the SL ligament is performed to confirm adequate tissue for repair. If there are not adequate tissues, alternative methods of treatment are undertaken and it is presumed that the patient likely had an acute-on-chronic injury.

SURGICAL PROCEDURE
Reduction and Ligament Repair

The torn SL ligament is identified; it is usually found to be torn from the scaphoid. The avulsion

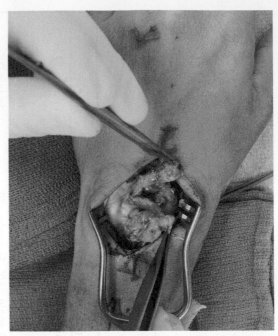

Fig. 2. Intraoperative demonstration of ulnar-based capsular flap.

site is debrided to create a base for ligament reattachment. This is done with a rongeur, a curette, and/or a small burr. A trial SL reduction is performed, often using 1.6-mm (0.062-inch) Kirschner wires (K-wires), one in the scaphoid and one in the lunate. This will allow the surgeon to assess where to place bone suture anchors and repair the ligament. Bone suture anchors are then placed and sutures passed in the corresponding location on the ligament, but not tied down (**Figs. 3** and **4**).

Final reduction of the SL joint is then performed. It is critical to rectify all alignment parameters: coronal shift (SL gap closed), sagittal DISI (radiolunate

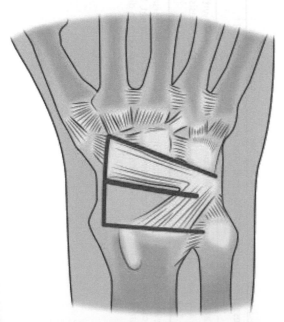

Fig. 1. Illustration of ulnar-based capsular flap. (*Courtesy of* Cynthia Conklin, CMI.)

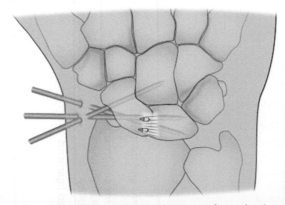

Fig. 3. Illustration of K-wire placement for reduction and initial suture anchor placement for SLIL repair. (*Courtesy of* Cynthia Conklin, CMI.)

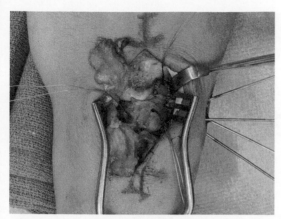

Fig. 4. Suture anchor placement for SLIL repair and capsulodesis.

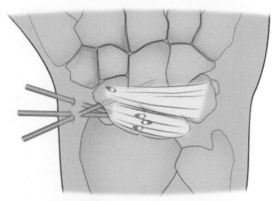

Fig. 5. Illustration of final SLIL repair and "double-dorsal" capsulodesis. (*Courtesy of* Cynthia Conklin, CMI.)

angle to 0°, capitolunate angle 0°, capitate head "covered" by the lunate, scaphoid de-flexed), dorsal translation (scaphoid returned back into its fossa), and scaphoid pronation. Once all reduction criteria are met (seen clinically and via fluoroscopic imaging), two 0.045 K-wires are placed in a divergent fashion across the SL joint and 1 to 2 wires placed across the scaphocapitate joint to secure reduction. These wires are placed through a small radial-sided incision to ensure protection of the superficial sensory radial nerve and the radial artery. Wires are also placed with the aid of a drill guide to avoid injury to the soft tissues. Wire placement is performed with the use of mini-C-arm fluoroscopy.

The preset sutures are then tied down in horizontal mattress configuration. The "double-dorsal" capsulodesis is then performed by tying down the proximal limb of the capsular flap to the scaphoid and lunate. The scaphoid side is tied to the existing bone suture anchor and the lunate side requires an additional bone suture anchor. The surrounding area on the lunate is prepared via curette to expose a few-millimeter area of bone for ligament to bone healing. The distal limb of the capsular flap is secured to the dorsal aspect of the distal pole of the scaphoid in a likewise manner via bone suture anchor for sagittal and rotational plane stability (**Figs. 5–7**).

Final Steps

The K-wires across the SL and scaphocapitate joints are cut beneath the skin and wounds closed. A dorsal and volar short-arm plaster splint is applied.

Immediate Postoperative Care

Finger range of motion (ROM) is instituted immediately postoperatively and continued throughout

the postoperative course. At 2 weeks postoperatively, the patient returns to the office for suture removal and placement of a fiberglass short-arm cast. Radiographs are obtained at this time to confirm reduction and appropriate hardware placement.

REHABILITATION AND RECOVERY

- At 6 weeks postoperatively, the short-arm cast is removed and replaced with a removable thermoplastic splint that the patient is instructed to wear at all times except when showering.

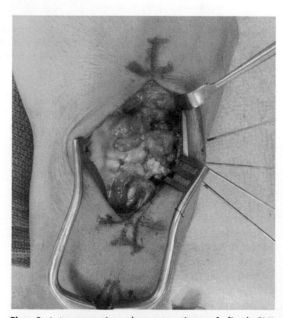

Fig. 6. Intraoperative demonstration of final SLIL repair and "double-dorsal" capsulodesis.

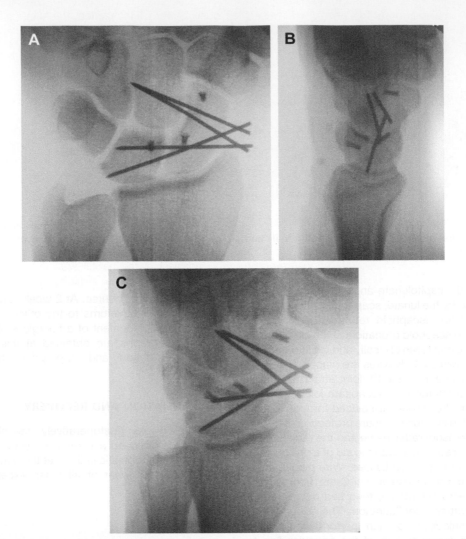

Fig. 7. (*A*) Intraoperative anteroposterior fluoroscopy demonstrating reduction and suture anchor placement. (*B*) Intraoperative lateral fluoroscopy demonstrating reduction and suture anchor placement. (*C*) Intraoperative oblique fluoroscopy demonstrating reduction and suture anchor placement.

- At 3 months postoperatively, K-wires are removed and the patient begins gentle ROM, initially beginning with dart-throwers range of motion (combined wrist extension/radial deviation and combined wrist flexion/ulnar deviation), as this is believed to put the scaphoid and lunate at minimal strain.[33,34] This is performed with the aid of a certified hand therapist.
- Between 4 and 4.5 months postoperatively, strengthening exercises are initiated.
- At 6 months postoperatively, the patient is released to unrestricted activity with the stipulation that there is a lifelong relative avoidance of extended wrist loading. We continue this restriction, as research has shown that in loaded wrist extension, there is a significant increase in SLIL strain, whereas there is minimal strain in the loaded neutral position.[35]

CLINICAL RESULTS IN THE LITERATURE

Acute treatment of SL ligament injury generally produces better results than treatment in the chronic phase. Rohman and colleagues[36] recently showed in a series of operatively treated SL injuries that wrists treated in the acute phase, of which many (16/24) had repair performed, had significantly lower failure rates than those treated in the chronic phase, as well as a tendency toward better QuickDASH scores and radiographic outcomes.

A review of the literature finds 3 independent studies that have performed suture anchor repair techniques similar to ours in a primarily acute setting with encouraging results (**Table 2**). Rosati and colleagues[37] in 2010 studied 18 patients retrospectively who had a mini-Mitek suture anchor repair. With an average follow-up of 32 months (range 9–68), 13 patients demonstrated excellent functional results and 3 demonstrated good results. There was loss of reduction in 2 cases. Bickert and colleagues[38] in 2000 performed 12 SLIL repairs with mini-Mitek suture anchors with an average follow-up of 19 months (range 8–27 months). They report 8 excellent or good functional results, a mean DASH (disabilities of the arm, shoulder, and hand score) score of 21, grip strength 81% of the uninjured side and ROM 78% of the uninjured side. In their cohort, they experienced 1 episode of re-dissociation (SL gap 5 mm).

The third report of acutely treated SLIL injuries with mini-Mitek suture anchor repair[39] also included a dorsal capsulodesis. The investigators followed 14 patients treated within 2 months of injury and 3 patients treated in a delayed fashion. Mean follow-up was 49 months (range 12–72 months). The investigators found an average 83 of 100 on the Green and O'Brien clinical grading system (93/100 for patients operated on within 2 months of injury), a mean SL angle of 49° (with a statistically better angle in the immediately treated group), and no SL gap. Only one of the early-treatment patients demonstrated degenerative changes on radiographs, whereas all of the delayed-treatment patients did. The investigators found good extension (87%) compared with the contralateral wrist, although significantly decreased flexion (70%), with statistically significant overall improvements in the earlier treatment group.

An additional article reports on SLIL repair in the acute setting using a transosseous suture technique.[40] In this report, 18 professional basketball players were treated (16 within 4–8 weeks of injury). Follow-up ranged from 16 to 180 months (average 62 months). Repair involved small drill holes for SLIL repair and dorsal capsulodesis. All patients rated good or excellent on a Mayo scale at follow-up. The SL angle averaged 62° and the SL gap averaged 2.5 mm postoperatively. Fifteen of the 18 patients were without evidence of degenerative changes on final radiographs (see **Table 2**).

In 2013, Chennagiri and Lindau[41] performed a review of management of SL instability in the absence of arthritis. Five articles in their review relate to open repair.[42–46] All of these articles included capsulodesis (one of which used tendon graft capsulodesis) and all types of instability (predynamic, dynamic, static, acute, and chronic) were included. Of these 5 articles, all were primarily (majority) chronic repairs rather than acute. Two articles used transosseous suture repair of the SLIL and 1 used suture anchor repair, 1 article reported on a combination of repair techniques and 1 did not specifically report the technique used to the repair the SLIL. Results of primarily chronic repair range from poor to excellent in these reports (**Table 3**).

In addition to the articles found in the Chennagiri and Lindau[41] review, another article[47] reported on chronic repair of SLIL injury. Here, 22 patients were treated with a transosseous suture technique in the chronic setting. Mean follow-up at 63 months showed most patients with excellent or good functional results and no signs of degenerative change was seen in 73%. There is, however, an 11% loss of grip strength and a loss of 19° of ROM (see **Table 3**).

Throughout these reports, complications of direct SLIL repair include superficial pin track infections, retained wire fragments, early pin removals, hardware migration, superficial radial nerve neuropraxias, chronic regional pain syndrome (CRPS), persistent ligamentous laxity, and iatrogenic cartilage injury.[32,36,44,48] Less frequent complications include scaphoid avascular necrosis[49] and lunate avascular necrosis.[38] Additionally, wrist stiffness is reported, particularly loss of wrist flexion, possibly due to concomitant dorsal capsulodesis.[32]

SPECIAL CASE SCENARIO: OPEN TREATMENT OF ACUTE SCAPHOLUNATE INSTABILITY IN DISTAL RADIUS FRACTURES

Rates of SL ligament injury in distal radius fractures range from 4.7% to 54.5% when diagnosed by arthroscopy.[50–56] Rates when diagnosed radiographically range from 13.3% to 29%.[57–62] Mudgal and Hastings suggest the mechanism of this combined injury can be attributed to a combination of tensile stress in ulnar deviation and axial (compression) stress in either radial or ulnar deviation.[63,64] Overall, intra-articular fractures are associated with higher rates of SL injury but SL injury can be found in extra-articular fractures as well.[50–54,57–60,62]

Diagnosis of these concomitant injuries can be difficult. In 1997, Richards and colleagues[54] evaluated 118 distal radius fractures arthroscopically and found that 60% of patients with SL injury did not demonstrate an SL gap greater than 2 mm on radiographs. In a 2008 study by Pliefke and colleagues,[65] radiographs correctly diagnosed 57% of arthroscopically diagnosed SL injuries (false negative in 18 of 42) and incorrectly diagnosed 1.7% (false positive in 1 of 42). Gradl and colleagues[66] report that radiographs provide

Table 2
Repair of acute SL injury

Author, Year	N	Time to Repair (Range)	Repair Type	Capsulodesis, Yes/No	Mean Follow-up (Range)	Results
Bickert et al,[38] 2000	12	41 d (no range)	Anchor	No	19 mo (8–27)	Mean DASH 21, Grip 81%, ROM 78%, 1 re-dissociation
Rosati et al,[37] 2010	18	10.5 d (2–21)	Anchor	No	32 mo (9–68)	16 excellent/good function, 2 losses of reduction
Minami et al,[39] 2003	17 (14 acute)	Acute <2 mo	Anchor	Yes	49 mo (12–72)	93/100 Green and O'Brien score, mean SL angle 49°, no SL gap, ROM 87% extension, 70% flexion, 13/14 no degenerative changes
Melone et al,[40] 2012	18 (16 acute)	Acute <2 mo	Transosseous	Yes	62 mo (16–180)	All good/excellent Mayo scores, average SL angle 62°, average SL gap 2.5 mm, 15/18 no degenerative changes

Abbreviations: DASH, disabilities of the arm, shoulder and hand score; ROM, range of motion; SL, scapholunate.
Data from Refs.[27,38–40]

Table 3
Repair of chronic SL injury

Author, Year	N	Time to Repair (Range)	Repair Type	Capsulodesis, Yes/No	Mean Follow-up (Range)	Results
Lavernia et al,[42] 1992	21	17 mo (1–84)	Transosseous	Yes (in 14)	33 mo (18–96)	Significant flexion loss (11.5°), equivalent grip, pain absent/minimal, 3/21 with degenerative changes
Pomerance,[44] 2006	17	22 wk (18–40)	Transosseous	Yes	66 mo (19–120)	Decline in clinical/radiographic parameters in patients with strenuous jobs
Wyrick et al,[46] 1998	17	3 mo (3 d–19 mo)	Anchor	Yes	30 mo (12–84)	Overall poor results: pain in all, 70% grip, 60% ROM, no change from injury to final radiographs
Saffar et al,[45] 1999	24	6.1 mo (0.25–36)	Both	Yes/No	27 mo (2–62)	Mean SL gap 3.7–5.3 mm, SL angle 58 deg, ROM/grip >75% contralateral side
Misra and Hales,[43] 2003	15	8.2 mo (7–14)	Unclear	Yes	22 mo (8–60)	13 good/excellent (Glickel/Millender), grip 58%, UD 53%, ext 62%, flex 49%
Schweizer and Steiger,[47] 2002	22	6 mo (1–35)	Transosseous	Yes (to proximal scaphoid)	63 mo (12–134)	18/22 excellent/good Green and O'Brien score, 10° flex loss, 9° ext loss, 11% grip loss, 6/22 degenerative changes

Grip % compared with contralateral, ROM %/degree compared with contralateral.
Abbreviations: ext, extension; flex, flexion; ROM, range of motion; SL, scapholunate; UD, ulnar deviation.
Data from Refs.[42–47]

69% sensitivity and 84% specificity in diagnosing SL dissociation when compared with intraoperative findings.

Routine arthroscopy as a diagnostic tool, however, is often not practical depending on the surgeon's practice. Recently, investigators have suggested alternative means of diagnosing these combined injuries. Suzuki and colleagues[67] in 2014 found that improved diagnostic accuracy can occur with analysis of the distal end of the SL joint on a central coronal CT slice with more than 2 mm indicating SL dissociation. Kwon and colleagues[68] described the utility of an intraoperative fluoroscopic carpal stretch test for identifying disruption of the proximal carpal row joint line. This showed a negative predictive value of 87% to rule out grade 3 or 4 SLIL tears in intra-articular distal radius fracture. An additional consideration in the diagnosis of these injuries, though, is the incidence of preexisting asymptomatic SL changes, particularly in the elderly,[69,70] which one needs to keep in mind in evaluating these injuries as well.

SL instability with associated distal radius fracture should be treated concurrently with distal radius fracture treatment. Geissler grade 3 changes may be treated with percutaneous pinning and Geissler grade 4 changes may be treated with open repair and dorsal capsulodesis. Studies have shown that failing to treat SL dissociation in patients with distal radius fracture leads to worse outcomes both clinically and radiographically.[56,58,59,61,62] Appropriate treatment, however, can provide good results. Peicha and colleagues[71] in 1999 performed arthroscopic-assisted K-wire fixation of Geissler grade 3 and 4 SL injuries with distal radius fracture with predominantly excellent or good results in patients at an average of 3 years of follow-up. Gradl and colleagues[72] recently reported that percutaneous or open pin fixation of grade 3 injuries and ligament repair of grade 4 injuries in addition to distal radius fracture treatment resulted in comparable outcomes to patients with an isolated distal radius fracture.

SUMMARY

Treatment of SL instability in the acute setting is paramount to prevent the long-term complications of DISI and SLAC wrist. Diagnosis is best made with clinical findings and positive static or stress radiographs. MRI and arthroscopy are valuable diagnostic adjuncts when necessary. In the acute setting, there is typically a repairable SLIL. Acute treatment of SL instability, therefore, involves direct SLIL ligament repair with a costabilizing dorsal capsulodesis. This has shown promising results in the literature. The modification of the dorsal capsulodesis to a "double-dorsal" capsulodesis confers additional strength to the SLIL repair.

ACKNOWLEDGMENTS

The authors thank Cynthia Conklin, CMI, for provision of surgical technique illustrations.

REFERENCES

1. Craigen MA, Stanley JK. Wrist kinematics. Row, column or both? J Hand Surg Br 1995;20(2):165–70.
2. Moojen TM, Snel JG, Ritt MJ, et al. In vivo analysis of carpal kinematics and comparative review of the literature. J Hand Surg Am 2003;28(1):81–7.
3. Garcia-Elias M. Carpal instability. In: Wolfe SW, Hotchkiss RN, Pederson WC, et al, editors. Green's operative hand surgery. Philadelphia: Elsevier; 2011. p. 465–522.
4. Manuel J, Moran SL. The diagnosis and treatment of scapholunate instability. Hand Clin 2010;26(1): 129–44.
5. Weber ER. Concepts governing the rotational shift of the intercalated segment of the carpus. Orthop Clin North Am 1984;15(2):193–207.
6. Wolfe SW, Neu C, Crisco JJ. In vivo scaphoid, lunate, and capitate kinematics in flexion and in extension. J Hand Surg Am 2000;25(5):860–9.
7. Ruby LK, An KN, Linscheid RL, et al. The effect of scapholunate ligament section on scapholunate motion. J Hand Surg Am 1987;12(5 Pt 1):767–71.
8. Short WH, Werner FW, Green JK, et al. Biomechanical evaluation of the ligamentous stabilizers of the scaphoid and lunate: part III. J Hand Surg Am 2007;32(3):297–309.
9. Berger RA, Bishop AT. A fiber-splitting capsulotomy technique for dorsal exposure of the wrist. Tech Hand Up Extrem Surg 1997;1:2–10.
10. Kuo CE, Wolfe SW. Scapholunate instability: current concepts in diagnosis and management. J Hand Surg Am 2008;33(6):998–1013.
11. Viegas SF, Yamaguchi S, Boyd NL, et al. The dorsal ligaments of the wrist: anatomy, mechanical properties, and function. J Hand Surg Am 1999; 24(3):456–68.
12. Mitsuyasu H, Patterson RM, Shah MA, et al. The role of the dorsal intercarpal ligament in dynamic and static scapholunate instability. J Hand Surg Am 2004;29(2):279–88.
13. Drewniany JJ, Palmer AK, Flatt AE. The scapho-trapezial ligament complex: an anatomic and biomechanical study. J Hand Surg Am 1985; 10(4):492–8.

14. Watson HK, Ashmead D 4th, Makhlouf MV. Examination of the scaphoid. J Hand Surg Am 1988;13(5): 657–60.

15. Watson HK, Weinzweig J, Zeppieri J. The natural progression of scaphoid instability. Hand Clin 1997;13(1):39–49.

16. Wolfe SW, Crisco JJ. Mechanical evaluation of the scaphoid shift test. J Hand Surg Am 1994;19(5): 762–8.

17. Linscheid RL, Dobyns JH, Beabout JW, et al. Traumatic instability of the wrist. Diagnosis, classification, and pathomechanics. J Bone Joint Surg Am 1972;54(8):1612–32.

18. Schimmerl-Metz SM, Metz VM, Totterman SM, et al. Radiologic measurement of the scapholunate joint: implications of biologic variation in scapholunate joint morphology. J Hand Surg Am 1999;24(6): 1237–44.

19. Lee SK, Desai H, Silver B, et al. Comparison of radiographic stress views for scapholunate dynamic instability in a cadaver model. J Hand Surg Am 2011;36(7):1149–57.

20. Lawand A, Foulkes GD. The "clenched pencil" view: a modified clenched fist scapholunate stress view. J Hand Surg Am 2003;28(3):414–8.

21. Kitay A, Wolfe SW. Scapholunate instability: current concepts in diagnosis and management. J Hand Surg Am 2012;37(10):2175–96.

22. Lee YH, Choi YR, Kim S, et al. Intrinsic ligament and triangular fibrocartilage complex (TFCC) tears of the wrist: comparison of isovolumetric 3D-THRIVE sequence MR arthrography and conventional MR image at 3 T. Magn Reson Imaging 2013;31(2):221–6.

23. Lee RK, Ng AW, Tong CS, et al. Intrinsic ligament and triangular fibrocartilage complex tears of the wrist: comparison of MDCT arthrography, conventional 3-T MRI, and MR arthrography. Skeletal Radiol 2013;42(9):1277–85.

24. Spaans AJ, Minnen Pv, Prins HJ, et al. The value of 3.0-tesla MRI in diagnosing scapholunate ligament injury. J Wrist Surg 2013;2(1):69–72.

25. Ruston J, Konan S, Rubinraut E, et al. Diagnostic accuracy of clinical examination and magnetic resonance imaging for common articular wrist pathology. Acta Orthop Belg 2013;79(4):375–80.

26. Abe Y, Katsube K, Tsue K, et al. Arthroscopic diagnosis of partial scapholunate ligament tears as a cause of radial sided wrist pain in patients with inconclusive x-ray and MRI findings. J Hand Surg Br 2006;31(4):419–25.

27. Morley J, Bidwell J, Bransby-Zachary M. A comparison of the findings of wrist arthroscopy and magnetic resonance imaging in the investigation of wrist pain. J Hand Surg Br 2001;26(6):544–6.

28. Hobby JL, Tom BD, Bearcroft PW, et al. Magnetic resonance imaging of the wrist: diagnostic performance statistics. Clin Radiol 2001;56(1):50–7.

29. Mayfield JK. Patterns of injury to carpal ligaments. A spectrum. Clin Orthop Relat Res 1984;(187):36–42.

30. Watson HK, Ballet FL. The SLAC wrist: scapholunate advanced collapse pattern of degenerative arthritis. J Hand Surg Am 1984;9(3):358–65.

31. Chim H, Moran SL. Wrist essentials: the diagnosis and management of scapholunate ligament injuries. Plast Reconstr Surg 2014;134(2):312e–22e.

32. Szabo RM. Scapholunate ligament repair with capsulodesis reinforcement. J Hand Surg Am 2008; 33(9):1645–54.

33. Werner FW, Green JK, Short WH, et al. Scaphoid and lunate motion during a wrist dart throw motion. J Hand Surg Am 2004;29(3):418–22.

34. Gardner MJ, Crisco JJ, Wolfe SW. Carpal kinematics. Hand Clin 2006;22(4):413–20.

35. Lee SK, Park J, Baskies M, et al. Differential strain of the axially loaded scapholunate interosseus ligament. J Hand Surg Am 2010;35(2):245–51.

36. Rohman EM, Agel J, Putnam MD, et al. Scapholunate interosseous ligament injuries: a retrospective review of treatment and outcomes in 82 wrists. J Hand Surg Am 2014;39(10):2020–6.

37. Rosati M, Parchi P, Cacianti M, et al. Treatment of acute scapholunate ligament injuries with bone anchor. Musculoskelet Surg 2010;94:25–32.

38. Bickert B, Sauerbier M, Germann G. Scapholunate ligament repair using the Mitek bone anchor. J Hand Surg Br 2000;25(2):188–92.

39. Minami A, Kato H, Iwasaki N. Treatment of scapholunate dissociation: ligamentous repair associated with modified dorsal capsulodesis. Hand Surg 2003;8(1):1–6.

40. Melone CP, Polatsch DB, Flink G, et al. Scapholunate interosseous ligament disruption in professional basketball players: treatment by direct repair and dorsal ligamentoplasty. Hand Clin 2012; 28:253–60.

41. Chennagiri RJ, Lindau TR. Assessment of scapholunate instability and review of evidence for management in the absence of arthritis. J Hand Surg Eur Vol 2013;38:727–38.

42. Lavernia CJ, Cohen MS, Taleisnik J. Treatment of scapholunate dissociation by ligamentous repair and capsulodesis. J Hand Surg Am 1992;17(2): 354–9.

43. Misra A, Hales P. Blatt's capsulodesis for chronic scapholunate instability. Acta Orthop Belg 2003; 69(3):233–8.

44. Pomerance J. Outcome after repair of the scapholunate interosseous ligament and dorsal capsulodesis for dynamic scapholunate instability due to trauma. J Hand Surg Am 2006;31(8):1380–6.

45. Saffar P, Sokolow C, Duclos L. Soft tissue stabilization in the management of chronic scapholunate instability without osteoarthritis. A 15-year series. Acta Orthop Belg 1999;65(4):424–33.

46. Wyrick JD, Youse BD, Kiefhaber TR. Scapholunate ligament repair and capsulodesis for the treatment of static scapholunate dissociation. J Hand Surg Br 1998;23(6):776–80.

47. Schweizer A, Steiger R. Long-term results after repair and augmentation ligamentoplasty of rotatory subluxation of the scaphoid. J Hand Surg Am 2002; 27(4):674–84.

48. Beredjiklian PK, Dugas J, Gerwin M. Primary repair of the scapholunate ligament. Tech Hand Up Extrem Surg 1998;2(4):269–73.

49. Berschback JC, Kalainov DM, Bednar MS. Osteonecrosis of the scaphoid after scapholunate interosseous ligament repair and dorsal capsulodesis: case report. J Hand Surg Am 2010;35(5):732–5.

50. Araf M, Mattar Junior R. Arthroscopic study of injuries in articular fractures of distal radius extremity. Acta Ortop Bras 2014;22(3):144–50.

51. Ogawa T, Tanaka T, Yanai T, et al. Analysis of soft tissue injuries associated with distal radius fractures. BMC Sports Sci Med Rehabil 2013;5(1):19.

52. Lindau T, Arner A, Hagber L. Intrarticular lesions in distal fractures of the radius in young adults. J Hand Surg Br 1997;22(5):638–43.

53. Geissler WB, Freeland AE, Savoie FH, et al. Intracarpal soft-tissue lesions associated with an intraarticular fracture of the distal end of the radius. J Bone Joint Surg Am 1996;78(3):357–65.

54. Richards RS, Bennett JD, Roth JH, et al. Arthroscopic diagnosis of intra-articular soft tissue injuries associated with distal radial fractures. J Hand Surg Am 1997;22(5):772–6.

55. Peicha G, Seibert FJ, Fellinger M, et al. Lesions of the scapholunate ligaments in acute wrist trauma–arthroscopic diagnosis and minimally invasive treatment. Knee Surg Sports Traumatol Arthrosc 1997; 5(3):176–83.

56. Forward DP, Lindau TR, Melsom DS. Intercarpal ligament injuries associated with fractures of the distal part of the radius. J Bone Joint Surg Am 2007; 89(11):2334–40.

57. Porter ML, Tillman RM. Pilon fractures of the wrist. Displaced intra-articular fractures of the distal radius. J Hand Surg Br 1992;17(1):63–8.

58. Gunal I, Ozaksoy D, Altay T, et al. Scapholunate dissociation associated with distal radius fractures. Eur J Orthop Surg Traumatol 2013;23(8):877–81.

59. Stoffelen D, De Mulder K, Broos P. The clinical importance of carpal instabilities following distal radial fractures. J Hand Surg Br 1998;23(4):512–6.

60. Tang JB. Carpal instability associated with fracture of the distal radius. Incidence, influencing factors and pathomechanics. Chin Med J (Engl) 1992; 105(9):758–65.

61. Tang JB, Shi D, Gu YQ, et al. Can cast immobilization successfully treat scapholunate dissociation associated with distal radius fractures? J Hand Surg Am 1996;21(4):583–90.

62. Laulan J, Bismuth JP. Intracarpal ligamentous lesions associated with fractures of the distal radius: outcome at one year. A prospective study of 95 cases. Acta Orthop Belg 1999;65:418–23.

63. Mudgal C, Hastings H. Scapho-lunate diastasis in fractures of the distal radius. Pathomechanics and treatment options. J Hand Surg Br 1993;18(6): 725–9.

64. Mudgal CS, Jones WA. Scapho-lunate diastasis: a component of fractures of the distal radius. J Hand Surg Br 1990;15(4):503–5.

65. Pliefke J, Stengel D, Rademacher G, et al. Diagnostic accuracy of plain radiographs and cineradiography in diagnosing traumatic scapholunate dissociation. Skeletal Radiol 2008;37(2):139–45.

66. Gradl G, Neuhaus V, Fuchsberger T, et al. Radiographic diagnosis of scapholunate dissociation among intra-articular fractures of the distal radius: interobserver reliability. J Hand Surg Am 2013; 38(9):1685–90.

67. Suzuki D, Ono H, Furuta K, et al. Comparison of scapholunate distance measurements on plain radiography and computed tomography for the diagnosis of scapholunate instability associated with distal radius fracture. J Orthop Sci 2014;19(3):465–70.

68. Kwon BC, Choi SJ, Song SY, et al. Modified carpal stretch test as a screening test for detection of scapholunate interosseous ligament injuries associated with distal radial fractures. J Bone Joint Surg Am 2011;93(9):855–62.

69. Rimington TR, Edwards SG, Lynch TS, et al. Intercarpal ligamentous laxity in cadaveric wrists. J Bone Joint Surg Br 2010;92(11):1600–5.

70. Akahane M, Ono H, Nakamura T, et al. Static scapholunate dissociation diagnosed by scapholunate gap view in wrists with or without distal radius fractures. Hand Surg 2002;7(2):191–5.

71. Peicha G, Seibert F, Fellinger M, et al. Midterm results of arthroscopic treatment of scapholunate ligament lesions associated with intra-articular distal radius fractures. Knee Surg Sports Traumatol Arthrosc 1999;7(5):327–33.

72. Gradl G, Pillukat T, Fuchsberger T, et al. The functional outcome of acute scapholunate ligament repair in patients with intraarticular distal radius fractures treated by internal fixation. Arch Orthop Trauma Surg 2013;133(9):1281–7.

Chronic Scapholunate Ligament Injury
Techniques in Repair and Reconstruction

Brett F. Michelotti, MD[a], Joshua M. Adkinson, MD[b],
Kevin C. Chung, MD, MS[c],*

KEYWORDS

- Wrist • Ligamentous injury • Scapholunate injury • Ligamentous reconstruction

KEY POINTS

- Scapholunate interosseous ligament injury exists as a spectrum of pathology that is best treated surgically after early recognition.
- Repair of the dorsal scapholunate ligament should be performed when possible.
- Decision to perform a direct reconstruction of the dorsal scapholunate ligament versus augmentation or reconstruction of the secondary scaphoid stabilizing ligaments depends on the presence or absence of rotatory subluxation of the scaphoid.
- Comparative studies suggest that all types of reconstruction for static scapholunate instability result in worsening of radiographic parameters and the development of arthrosis, although not all patients require a salvage operation.
- A salvage operation, such as a partial wrist fusion, should be considered when there is clinical and radiographic evidence of wrist arthritis.

INTRODUCTION

Although the true incidence of scapholunate interosseous ligament (SLIL) injury is unknown, a study by Lee and colleagues[1] found that 35% of cadaveric wrists had some degree of SL tear. Of those wrists with SLIL injury, 29% had evidence of arthrosis. Early recognition and treatment of these injuries can delay or prevent the onset of arthritis.

Soft tissue repair or reconstruction of the SLIL presents a difficult problem, with varied clinical results, long-term durability, and wrist function.

Many operative techniques have been developed for different stages along the injury spectrum. Although primary healing of the SLIL likely provides the best opportunity for maintenance of normal carpal kinematics and prevention of wrist arthroses, several operative techniques have been developed in an attempt to prevent rotatory subluxation of the scaphoid and the subsequent development of wrist arthritis (**Box 1**).

The goal of this article is to detail treatment options for SLIL injury across the spectrum of

Supported in part by grants from the National Institute on Aging and National Institute of Arthritis and Musculoskeletal and Skin Diseases (R01 AR062066, 2R01 AR047328-06), and a Midcareer Investigator Award in Patient-Oriented Research (K24 AR053120) (to Dr K.C. Chung).
Conflicts of Interest: The authors have no conflicts of interest.
Financial Disclosure: None.
[a] Section of Plastic Surgery, Department of Surgery, University of Michigan Health System, 2130 Taubman Center, SPC 5340, 1500 East Medical Center Drive, Ann Arbor, MI 48109-5340, USA; [b] Section of Plastic Surgery, Department of Surgery, Northwestern University Feinberg School of Medicine, NMH/Galter Room 3-150, 251 E Huron, Chicago, IL 60611, USA; [c] Section of Plastic Surgery, University of Michigan Medical School, University of Michigan Health System, 2130 Taubman Center, SPC 5340, 1500 East Medical Center Drive, Ann Arbor, MI 48109-5340, USA
* Corresponding author.
E-mail address: kecchung@umich.edu

hand.theclinics.com

Box 1
Results from the ideal scapholunate ligament repair or reconstruction

1. Healing of the dorsal scapholunate interosseus ligament (SLIL)

2. Maintenance of reduction of the scapholunate (SL) interval and preservation of the normal anatomic relationships of the carpus

3. Prevention of the biomechanical alteration that can lead to progressive arthrosis

4. Limited morbidity to the uninjured structures of the wrist

pathology with a particular emphasis on chronic SL repair and reconstruction. We also aim to present new techniques and outcomes data.

ANATOMY AND CARPAL KINEMATICS

The proximal carpal row is composed of the scaphoid, lunate, triquetrum, and pisiform, a sesamoid bone that is enveloped by the flexor carpi ulnaris. The mobility of the proximal row permits wrist flexion, extension, radial deviation, and ulnar deviation, as well as thumb opposition and pronation. Dense interosseous ligaments connect the bones of the proximal carpal row, and these include the SLIL and the lunotriquetral interosseous ligament; these are the primary stabilizers of the carpus (**Fig. 1**). The SLIL is composed of palmar, proximal, and dorsal fibers (**Fig. 2**). The strongest part of the ligament runs within the deep portion of the wrist capsule and links the dorsal scaphoid and lunate. The dorsal portion of the ligament has an average yield strength of 260 N. The palmar portion of the ligament contains obliquely oriented fibers that are weaker (118 N yield strength) but permit more rotation around the lunate and play less of a role in stability than the stronger dorsal ligament. The proximal membranous portion of the ligament (63 N yield strength) does not play a role in stabilization and often appears perforated in older individuals, but this is not a true indication of SLIL instability.[2]

Secondary stabilizers of the carpus include both bony constraints and the extrinsic wrist ligaments. The dorsal extrinsic ligaments include the dorsal radiocarpal ligament (DRC) and the dorsal intercarpal ligament (DIC). The DRC begins on the distal radius, travels across and sends attachments to the lunate before terminating on the dorsal triquetrum. The DIC spans from the triquetrum to the scaphoid with attachments to the lunate, capitate, trapezium, and trapezoid. The DRC and DIC have become important anatomic landmarks

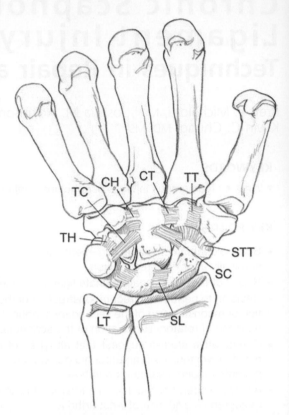

Fig. 1. Intrinsic ligaments of the wrist. CH, capitohamate; CT, capitotrapeziod; LT, lunotriquetral; SC, scaphocapitate; SL, scapholunate; STT, scapho-trapezium-trapezoid; TC, triquetrocapitate; TH, triquetrohamate; TT, trapezium-trapezoid ligaments.

for the ligament-sparing approach to the wrist and provide tissue in several techniques that augment SLIL repair or reconstruction.[2]

The palmar extrinsic and intrinsic ligaments of importance in SL destabilization include the radioscaphocapitate ligament (RSC), the long and short radiolunate ligaments, and the scaphotrapezoid and scaphotrapezial ligaments (STT). Extrinsic ligaments originating from the distal ulna include the ulnolunate, lunocapitate, and ulnotriquetral ligaments. These ligaments are not as important in maintaining proper carpal alignment following intercarpal ligamentous injury (**Fig. 3**).

The interosseous ligaments of the proximal carpal row lead to predictable anatomic changes when different forces are exerted across the wrist. With radial deviation, the scaphoid moves into a flexed position and pulls the lunate into slight flexion. With ulnar deviation, the geometry of the hamate/triquetral articulation pushes the triquetrum into extension, whereas the dense attachments of the lunotriquetral ligament pull the lunate and scaphoid into slight extension. When the ligamentous attachments are disrupted and

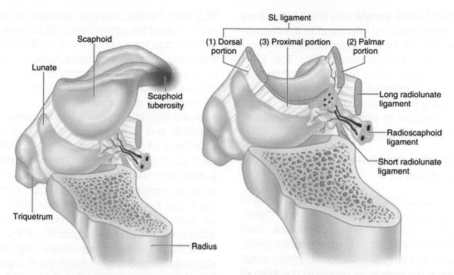

Fig. 2. SLIL. (*From* Sebastin SJ, Ono S, Chung KC. Scapholunate ligament reconstruction using a flexor carpi radialis tendon graft. In: Chung KC, editor. Operative techniques: hand and wrist surgery. 2nd edition. Philadelphia: Elsevier Saunders; 2012. p. 679; with permission.)

the secondary stabilizers are either acutely torn or attenuated, the proximal carpal row become unlinked and dissociative carpal instability occurs. When intercarpal ligamentous injuries are identified before the onset of wrist arthritis, soft tissue reconstructive procedures can be performed to restore some form of carpal alignment in an attempt to prevent or delay the progression of painful degenerative changes.

Gardner and colleagues[3] have performed extensive research detailing the in vivo relationships of the carpus during normal wrist motion, flexion/extension, the radial/extended to flexed/ulnarly deviated arc of the dart-throwers motion (DTM), and the extremes of the flexion and extension.[4–6] This in vivo 3-dimensional computed tomography scan evaluation documented the position of the carpus with axial loading in extremes of motion

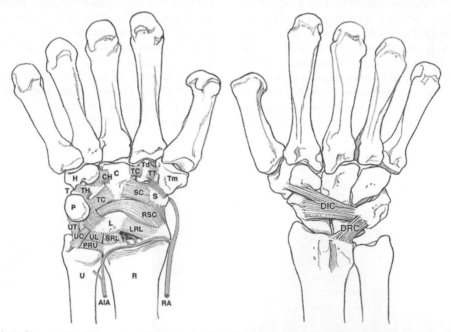

Fig. 3. Extrinsic ligaments of the wrist. AIA, anterior interosseous artery; C, capitate; DIC, dorsal intercarpal ligament; DRC, Dorsal radiocarpal ligament; H, hamate; LRL, long radiolunate; P, pisiform; PRU, palmar radioulnar; R, radius; RA, radial artery; RSC, Radioscaphocapitate; S, scaphoid; SRL, short radiolunate; T, triquetrum; Td, trapezoid; Tm, trapezium; U, ulna; UC, ulnocapitate; UL, ulnolunate; UT, ulnotriquetral ligament.

and provided further insight into the ligamentous and bony constraints that often lead to the characteristic patterns of both ligamentous and combined bony and ligamentous injury. The DTM confers a degree of agility and fluidity when performing daily and recreational tasks but also may provide stability by reducing midcarpal motion.[7,8] This can be applied to principles of rehabilitation after repair of wrist ligamentous injuries.

CLASSIFICATION OF SCAPHOLUNATE LIGAMENT INJURY

Injury to the SL ligament is most often the result of trauma caused by a fall onto an outstretched hand. This may be associated with fractures of the distal radius and greater and lesser arc perilunate injuries. Although less common, SLIL dissociation may result from attritional degeneration owing to rheumatoid arthritis, Kienböck disease, or pseudogout.[9–13]

SLIL injuries present along a spectrum of disease. Several classification systems exist to guide treatment. The simplest way to conceptualize SLIL injury is to designate the injury pattern into 1 of 5 instability groups: predynamic, dynamic, static-reducible, static-irreducible, and SL advanced collapse (SLAC). Predynamic instability is the result of a partially torn or attenuated ligament and can present as wrist pain, exacerbated by heavy lifting. This stage has normal radiograph findings, although the diagnosis can be confirmed arthroscopically.[14] Dynamic instability is best diagnosed with standard clenched-fist radiographs; this maneuver results in the greatest widening of the SL interval.[15] Originally described by Foulkes, the "clenched pencil" radiograph requires bilateral forearm pronation, while grasping of a pencil with a clenched fist. This maneuver promotes wrist ulnar deviation and opposition of the first web space, while accentuating a near complete or complete SLIL tear. Further, this view allows for simultaneous evaluation of the contralateral SL interval within the same image for comparison (**Fig. 4**). With dynamic instability, posterior-anterior, oblique, and lateral radiographs will show normal anatomic alignment of the proximal row from the intact secondary stabilizers of the scaphoid.

Static instability results from a complete tear of the SLIL and attenuation or tearing of secondary stabilizers of the scaphoid (ie, STT, RSC, and/or DIC). Carpal malalignment can be observed with a standard radiographic evaluation of the wrist without increasing the axial load. Chronicity of the injury becomes important in static instability as repair or reconstruction versus a salvage operation depends on the reducibility of the scaphoid.

Although the temporal relationship between SL dissociation and onset of arthritis is unknown, carpal malalignment and altered biomechanics can lead to a predictable and sequential pattern of disease. Standard radiographs may reveal radial styloid (stage 1), radioscaphoid (stage 2), scaphocapitate (stage 3) to pancarpal (stage 4), or SLAC changes. SLAC is considered a contraindication for SL soft tissue reconstruction because of advanced articular wear.

DIAGNOSIS

Diagnosis of SLIL injury starts with a history of dorsal wrist pain exacerbated by lifting or axial loading and should prompt careful physical examination of the SL interval. Palpation distal to the Lister tubercle and the Watson scaphoid shift test may elicit pain or dorsal translation of the scaphoid. Standard radiographs may demonstrate static SL injury, including greater than 3-mm gap in the SL interval (Terry Thomas sign) (**Fig. 5**A), scaphoid ring sign (flexion of the scaphoid resulting in the distal pole projecting through the proximal pole),

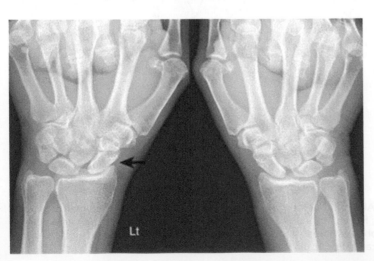

Fig. 4. Clenched-fist maneuver. The *arrow* illustrates arthritis changes involving the radial styloid and radioscaphoid joint. Lt, left. (*From* Sebastin SJ, Ono S, Chung KC. Scapholunate ligament reconstruction using a flexor carpi radialis tendon graft. In: Chung KC, editor. Operative techniques: hand and wrist surgery. 2nd edition. Philadelphia: Elsevier Saunders; 2012. p. 679; with permission.)

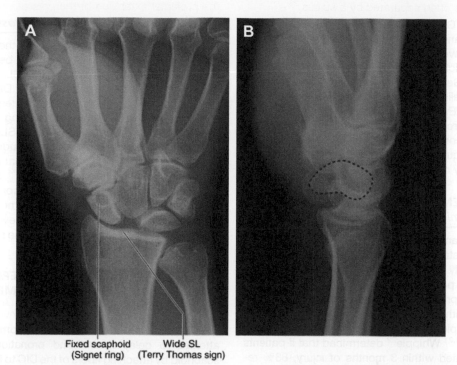

Fixed scaphoid   Wide SL
(Signet ring)   (Terry Thomas sign)

Fig. 5. (*A*) Scaphoid ring sign and Terry Thomas sign. (*B*) Lateral radiograph demonstrating an increased SL angle. (*From* Sebastin SJ, Ono S, Chung KC. Scapholunate ligament reconstruction using a flexor carpi radialis tendon graft. In: Chung KC, editor. Operative techniques: hand and wrist surgery. 2nd edition. Philadelphia: Elsevier Saunders; 2012. p. 677; with permission.)

or a disruption of Gilula arcs representing malalignment of the carpus. The SL angle may be greater than 60° (normally between 30° and 60°), resulting from flexion of the scaphoid and extension of the lunate leading to the characteristic dorsal intercalated segment instability (DISI) deformity (see **Fig. 5**B). Rhee and colleagues[16] determined that the bony morphology of the lunate might play a role in preventing the DISI deformity. Preoperative radiographs in a cohort of 58 patients who

underwent repair or reconstruction of the SLIL were examined retrospectively. Patients with a type II lunate, or the presence of a medial hamate facet, were less likely to develop DISI deformity.

Predynamic injury may be identified only by arthroscopic evaluation. Geissler developed a classification system for SLIL injuries based on intraoperative arthroscopic evaluation (**Table 1**). Grades I to III of the Geissler classification system represent predynamic instability or partial injury to

Table 1
Geissler arthroscopic classification of carpal interosseous ligament tears

Grade	Description
I	Attenuation and hemorrhage of interosseous ligament seen from radiocarpal joint, with no step-off present as seen from midcarpal joint
II	Attenuation and hemorrhage of interosseous ligament seen from radiocarpal joint, with step-off seen through midcarpal joint; the probe can be placed between the scaphoid and lunate
III	Incongruence or step-off is seen between the scaphoid and the lunate from both the radiocarpal and midcarpal portals; the probe can be placed and freely rotated between the scaphoid and lunate
IV	Incongruence or step-off is seen between the scaphoid and lunate from both the radiocarpal and midcarpal portals; gross instability is noted, and the 2.7-mm arthroscope may be passed through the gap between the scaphoid and lunate

Adapted from Geissler WB, Freeland AE, Savoie FH, et al. Intracarpal soft-tissue lesions associated with an intra-articular fracture of the distal end of the radius. J Bone Joint Surg Am 1996;78(3):357–65.

the SLIL. Grade IV represents gross instability of the SLIL and dynamic carpal instability.

Most investigators agree that 6 weeks is the demarcation between acute and chronic SLIL injuries.[17] Generally speaking, SLIL injuries have a better healing potential if treated early with direct repair.[17] Even with early detection and direct repair, chronic instability may occur; this requires SLIL reconstruction. Ligament reconstruction also is required if the dorsal SLIL is not amenable to primary repair.

TREATMENT
Predynamic Instability

Geissler and others[14,18,19] suggest that predynamic instability (Geissler grades I–III) can be adequately treated with arthroscopic management and percutaneous pinning of the SL interval. Chronic predynamic instability also has been treated with selective proprioceptive rehabilitation, arthroscopic debridement, or capsular shrinkage (Box 2).[20,21] Whipple[22] determined that if patients were treated within 3 months of injury, 83% remained symptom free and maintained their reduction in up to 7-year follow-up.

Box 2
Operative techniques based on type of instability and condition of remaining SL ligament

Predynamic instability

- Arthroscopic debridement, percutaneous pinning of SL interval
- Proprioceptive rehabilitation

Dynamic instability, direct repair possible

- Dorsal SLIL repair
- Dorsal SLIL + capsulodesis

Dynamic instability, direct repair not possible

- Ligamentous reconstruction from the dorsal intercarpal ligament
- Bone-tissue-bone graft
- Capsulodesis
- Reduction and association of the scaphoid and lunate
- Arthroscopic-assisted ligamentoplasty

Static, reducible instability

- Modified-Brunelli 3-ligament tenodesis
- Four-ligament tenodesis
- Scapholunotriquetral tenodesis
- Scapholunate axis method (SLAM)

Dynamic Instability, Direct Repair Possible

When there is complete disruption of the SL ligament (Geissler IV), direct repair should be attempted. With dynamic instability, the SL angle is preserved and there is no evidence of DISI deformity because the secondary stabilizers of the scaphoid are intact. Although repairing both the palmar and dorsal components of the SLIL seems anatomically appropriate, recent studies have shown that the dorsal ligament is all that is necessary to maintain carpal alignment.[2,23,24] There are no data to suggest that a complex reconstruction or ligamentoplasty should be performed at this stage in the absence of radiographic evidence of failure of the secondary stabilizers of the scaphoid.

OPERATIVE TECHNIQUE (DIRECT REPAIR WITH DORSAL INTERCARPAL LIGAMENT CAPSULODESIS)

Direct repair with capsulodesis is performed in an attempt to delay flexion and pronation of the scaphoid by attaching fibers of the DIC to its dorsal, distal pole. The wrist is approached through a dorsal longitudinal incision over the Lister tubercle. Two extensor retinacular flaps are elevated in stair-step fashion, exposing the third and fourth extensor compartments. A ligament-sparing approach to the wrist capsule is performed following the fibers of the DRC and DIC ligaments (Fig. 6).[25] The incision then begins at the radial styloid and follows the oblique fibers of the DRC across the lunate fossa onto the dorsal cortex of the triquetrum. The transverse portion of the incision should begin at the STT joint, course across the capitate, and join the oblique incision over the dorsal triquetrum. This radially based flap provides direct visualization of the SL interval. Preservation of the distal half of the DIC is essential if a dorsal capsulodesis will be performed to augment the repair.

The fibers of dorsal ligament may be attenuated or directly avulsed with a bony fragment still attached. If the ligament ends have been avulsed and can be reapproximated with reasonable repair strength, direct suture repair should be performed. Where a bony fragment has been avulsed from the dorsal cortex, the bone should be replaced and fixated with transosseous wires or suture anchors. The direct repair should be augmented with Kirschner-wire (K-wire) fixation of the SL and scaphocapitate joints and dorsal capsulodesis should also be considered. In chronic SL injury, direct repair may not be possible and therefore the patient should be prepared for a ligamentous reconstruction.[26]

Although more commonly used in chronic, static SL dissociation, the DIC capsulodesis may be

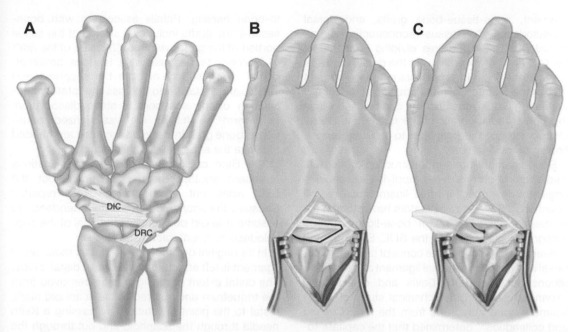

Fig. 6. Ligament-sparing approach to the wrist. (*A*) Orientation of DRC and DIC. (*B*) Radial-sided capsular flap markings. (*C*) Elevation of a ligament-sparing capsular flap to expose the carpal bones. (*From* Sebastin SJ, Ono S, Chung KC. Scapholunate ligament reconstruction using a flexor carpi radialis tendon graft. In: Chung KC, editor. Operative techniques: hand and wrist surgery. 2nd edition. Philadelphia: Elsevier Saunders; 2012. p. 681; with permission.)

used to augment the repair if the ligament does not appear healthy or the strength of the repair is questionable. Originally described as detachment of the radial-sided fibers of the DIC from the scaphoid, trapezium, and trapezoid, the distal half of the DIC can be detached following a ligament-sparing approach to the wrist.[27,28]

After ensuring reduction of the scaphoid and lunate, a trough is created on the dorsal aspect of the scaphoid, distal to its axis of rotation, to act as a dorsal force opposing flexion of the distal pole. A suture anchor is placed within the bony trough and the radial side of the transected DIC can be tied down, into the trough, to augment the direct ligamentous repair.

Melone and colleagues[29] demonstrated that direct repair of the SLIL combined with dorsal ligamentoplasty can be performed in high-demand athletes with durable results. Surgery was performed at 1 week to 18 weeks from the time of injury and included direct SLIL repair with sutures passed through drill holes on the dorsal/ulnar aspect of the scaphoid augmented with the proximal portion of the DIC. With an average follow-up of 5 years, Mayo Wrist Scores were good or excellent (average 85), with a near-normal SL angle (62°) and SL gap (2.5 mm). Three of the 25 patients demonstrated radiographic evidence of symptomatic arthrosis at follow-up of more than 5 years.

Gajendran and colleagues[30] reported 7-year follow-up of patients who had direct repair of an SLIL injury supported with DIC capsulodesis. The investigators determined that 50% of patients developed radiographic signs of arthrosis, although subjective scores of function and patient satisfaction remained reasonably high.

Pooled data from several series in which investigators treated SL dissociation with direct ligamentous repair suggested that, at 3-year follow-up, most patients demonstrated reduced pain (70%) and regained grip strength and motion as compared with the contralateral side (80% strength, 70% motion). These data also suggest that high-demand patients are at a higher risk of developing radiographic changes associated with SLAC arthritis.[26,31–33] One study suggested that at 30-month follow-up, all 17 patients had persistent pain and the final SL angle was no different from the preoperative value (78° vs 72°, $P > .05$). These data suggest that direct repair with DIC augmentation fails to prevent rotatory collapse of the scaphoid and eventual progression of arthritis.[33]

Dynamic Instability, Direct Repair Not Possible

Several methods of reconstruction are available for patients with a dynamic instability, where direct repair is not possible. These include the use of adjacent tissues to reconstruct the dorsal SLIL ligament, bone-tissue-bone grafts, and dorsal capsulodeses. Soft tissue reconstruction of the dorsal SLIL often requires dividing remnants of the DIC or DRC by preserving the dorsal triquetral attachments, and repositioning the ligament across the SL interval in the position of a normally appearing SLIL. Bone anchors can be used within the dorsal radial corner of the lunate and dorsal ulnar corner of the scaphoid to facilitate repositioning of the ligament.[23]

Bone-ligament-bone reconstruction of the SLIL also should be considered, applying a technique originally described in knee ligamentous reconstruction.[34] Several investigators have studied the biomechanical potential of bone-ligament-bone autograft replacement of the SLIL. Svoboda and colleagues[35] described the concept of using metatarsal and dorsal metatarsal ligament as a means to reconstruct the SLIL. Davis and colleagues[36] expanded on the biomechanical study of bone-ligament-bone autografts from the foot. Cuenod and colleagues[37] determined that the capitate-to-trapezoid ligament more closely resembled the stiffness and failure load of the dorsal SLIL but the trapezoid to second metacarpal ligament was stronger and also could be used as a potential donor. The third metacarpal to capitate ligament or a segment of bone and retinaculum from the region of the Lister tubercle also can be used.[38–44]

Delayed graft healing and pullout from the scaphoid and lunate are complications associated with bone-tissue-bone reconstruction. Because of these complications, thought to be attributed to failure of osseous ingrowth, a vascularized graft of third metacarpal-capitate, based on the radial-sided intermetacarpal artery was designed.[45] This artery can be dissected proximally to the radial artery to provide sufficient length on mobilization and inset.

Long-term results of the distal radius bone-ligament-bone reconstruction described by Soong and colleagues[42] suggest that, on average, patients will go on to develop radioscaphoid arthritis, widening of the SL interval, and a decrease in wrist flexion and extension. Three of 6 patients who presented for long-term follow-up (mean follow-up 11.9 years) required total or partial wrist arthrodesis because of persistent pain and worsening wrist function. Intraoperative examination during these salvage procedures revealed one patient with an intact reconstruction and progressive arthritis, one patient with no graft remaining, and a third patient with partial graft remaining.

Bone-tissue-bone reconstruction is similar in both compliance and failure strength when compared with the dorsal SLIL.[37,40] Proponents of this technique suggest that bone-to-bone healing may be more predictable than ligament-to-bone healing. Pitfalls associated with bone-tissue-bone grafts include (1) stretch of the tissue portion of the graft over time, (2) failure of the graft to incorporate because of a tenuous proximal-dorsal blood supply of both the scaphoid and lunate, and (3) failure to address the rotatory subluxation of the scaphoid in static dissociation. Long-term results of the vascularized bone-tissue-bone graft in static dissociation are needed to prove the superiority of this technique.

The Blatt capsulodesis and its modifications represent another method to reconstruct the SLIL when not amenable to direct repair.[46] Because the scaphoid has a natural tendency to assume a flexed position, it is the goal of the capsulodesis to counteract these forces.

In its original description, the dorsal radiocarpal ligament is left attached to the dorsal distal radius. The distal extent of the ligament is removed from the triquetrum and sutured to the scaphoid neck, distal to the point of rotation, by passing a Keith needle through the scaphoid and out through the thenar skin where the sutures are tied over a button. Modifications of the technique have been described in which half of the dorsal intercarpal ligament is used and is either passed across the radiocarpal joint (Linscheid) or attached to the distal pole of the scaphoid without crossing the radiocarpal joint (Galendran).[23] Berger described a capsulodesis technique in which a strip of the DIC is detached from the triquetrum and sutured to the dorsal-proximal corner of the lunate after reduction of the scaphoid[25] (Fig. 7). Moran and

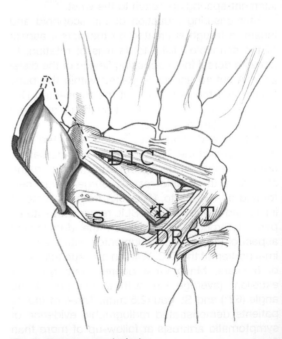

Fig. 7. Berger capsulodesis.

colleagues[47] then compared outcomes of the Berger-type capsulodesis with the modified-Brunelli tenodesis (MBT) in patients with chronic SL instability; no difference in grip strength, range of motion, or Mayo wrist scores were noted overall, or with cohort comparison of patients with dynamic or static dissociation.

Reduction and association of the scaphoid and lunate (RASL) can be performed for dynamic or static instability in which the ligament is not amenable to repair.[48] As originally described by Rosenwasser,[48] the cartilage is removed from both the scaphoid and lunate within the SL interval, and a headless compression screw is passed from the scaphoid waist to the proximal-ulnar corner of the lunate. When performed correctly, a fibrous union between the scaphoid and lunate occurs. The RASL procedure also can be performed arthroscopically, although there are reports of destruction of the scaphoid or lunate requiring subsequent screw removal.[49–51]

Larson and Stern[52] recently published short-term clinical and radiographic outcomes in which the RASL procedure resulted in early loss of reduction of the scaphoid and lunate and gapping of the SL interval. The RASL procedure also has been associated with avascular necrosis of the scaphoid.[53] If this procedure is attempted, all cartilage on the articular surfaces of the SL interval must be removed to bleeding cancellous bone to optimize the potential for fibrous union and to minimize motion across the joint that could lead to further destruction of the scaphoid or lunate.

Corella and colleagues[54,55] recently described the arthroscopically assisted ligamentoplasty for dynamic or easily reducible static instability. Reduction and maintenance of the SL interval is achieved by arthroscopically passing a slip of flexor carpi radialis (FCR) through the scaphoid and the lunate (dorsal to volar) to reconstruct both the dorsal and volar portion of the SL ligament. The investigators contend that open approaches damage the soft tissues and perhaps disrupt the dorsal secondary stabilizers of the scaphoid. Follow-up data are needed to confirm durability and satisfactory long-term outcomes after this approach.

Static-Reducible Instability

In this stage, the secondary stabilizing ligaments of the scaphoid have failed and the scaphoid has assumed a flexed, pronated posture. Important considerations at this stage of disease are (1) the reducibility of the scaphoid, and (2) the absence of the cartilage degeneration. An irreducible

scaphoid or the radiographic evidence of wrist arthritis should prompt consideration of a salvage procedure such as a partial wrist fusion.

Because the secondary stabilizers have been attenuated, SLIL reconstruction with or without dorsal capsulodesis tends to have less favorable outcomes when attempted for static dissociation as compared with reconstruction of the ligament during the dynamic stage of disease.[42] Tendon grafts have become an attractive option for treating static instability without evidence of arthritis. This technique has been described with several modifications since its original description. With the goal of preventing the degeneration of cartilage associated with altered wrist kinematics, various investigators have described the use of the extensor carpi radialis brevis (ECRB) and FCR to address scaphoid and lunate malalignment.[23,56]

The initial Brunelli tenodesis was well tolerated, as most patients were able to return to work with recovery of grip strength and absence of pain. Case series reported an average loss of wrist flexion of 45% as compared with the contralateral side.[56] For this reason, alteration of the technique led to the MBT, in which the FCR is not sutured to the distal radius, but instead anchored to the dorsal cortex of the lunate,[57] or passed through the dorsal radiocarpal ligament and anchored to the lunate or both the scaphoid and lunate **(Fig. 8)**.[58–60]

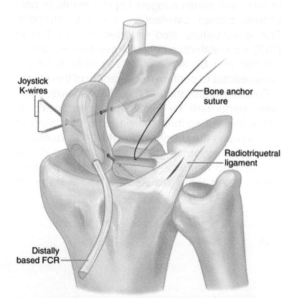

Fig. 8. Tendon reconstruction of the SLIL (Brunelli and modifications). (*From* Sebastin SJ, Ono S, Chung KC. Scapholunate ligament reconstruction using a flexor carpi radialis tendon graft. In: Chung KC, editor. Operative techniques: hand and wrist surgery. 2nd edition. Philadelphia: Elsevier Saunders; 2012. p. 685; with permission.)

Chabas and colleagues[61] reported outcomes of 19 patients who underwent MBT with average follow-up of 37 months (range 12–60 months). Fifteen patients had no or mild pain and 4 had constant pain. Wrist flexion and extension were reduced as compared with the contralateral side (average 41° flexion, average 50° extension). Static SL gap was 3.2 mm on average and one patient in the cohort went on to develop SLAC arthritis.

Nienstedt[62] recently published long-term follow-up (average 13.8 years) on a small series of patients with static, reducible SL injury treated with the MBT 3-ligament tenodesis (TLT). Green and O'Brien functional scores were excellent or good in 7 of 8 patients. At final follow-up, Disabilities of Arm, Shoulder and Hand scores (DASH) and Mayo wrist scores were 9 and 83, respectively. Total wrist motion and grip strength were maintained, averaging 85% of the contralateral side. Six of 8 patients were pain free, SL gap was maintained at an average of 2.8 mm, and the final SL angle averaged 63° at final follow-up. One patient in this cohort went on to develop SLAC arthritis.[62]

Bain and colleagues[59] further modified the MBT by using the FCR to reinforce the DIC, thereby creating a quad-ligament tenodesis. After passing the FCR through the DRC over the triquetrum, the tendon is sutured to the dorsal, distal cortex of the scaphoid to augment the DIC. Early clinical results of this case series suggest improvements in pain scores, patient satisfaction, and grip strength. The investigators also reported loss of flexion (70% contralateral side), and average SL gap of 3.0 mm and SL angle of 71°. Long-term follow-up is needed to confirm the durability of this repair.

Further modification of the MBT technique has been performed by Ross and colleagues[63] in which they described the passage of a strip of FCR through the scaphoid, lunate, and triquetrum. The distal aspect is then sutured to the dorsal scaphoid to reinforce the dorsal intercarpal ligament. Short-term results (at an average of

14 months) show maintenance of a reduced SL angle and gap (57° and 1.6 mm, respectively) in 11 patients. With this scapholunotriquetral transosseous tenodesis (SLT tenodesis), QuickDASH, Patient-related Wrist Evaluation scores, and grip strength all improved after surgery. Flexion/extension total range of motion decreased similar to reports of the Garcia-Elias modification (102° vs 103°). In a cadaver model, the SLT tenodesis performed as well as the MBT in maintaining normal anatomic parameters of the SL interval.[64]

The SL-axis method (SLAM) is a novel technique for reconstruction of the SL ligament. The SL interval is approached dorsally and a separate incision is made longitudinally over the anatomic snuff box. After reduction of scaphoid and lunate is ensured, a C-shaped guide is used to place a K-wire from the radial-sided waist of the scaphoid to the proximal-ulnar corner of the lunate, along the mid-axis. A second K-wire is used to maintain the position of the carpus during drilling. A cannulated step-drill (2.85 and 3.78 mm) is then used along the length of the guide wire. The tendon graft is secured within the lunate with a graft anchor, and an interference screw is placed within the drill hole on the radial side of the scaphoid (**Fig. 9**).

Biomechanical analysis in a cadaver model demonstrated that the SLAM maintained normal anatomic relationships of the SL interval and correction of the SL angle better than the commonly used Blatt capsulodesis and MBT.[65] Although results of cadaveric studies are not always realized in clinical practice, these biomechanical data indicate that the placement of a tendon graft along the axis of rotation of the SL interval compares favorably with the aforementioned techniques that are currently used. The advantage of the SLAM over the RASL procedure is that the tendon graft permits motion about the scaphoid and lunate in more than one plane, and this theoretically reduces the risk of cortical disruption.

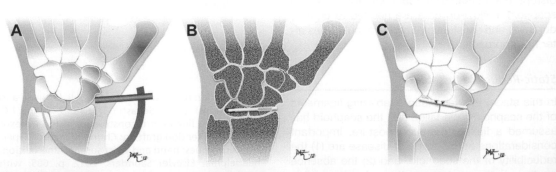

Fig. 9. (A–C) SLAM.

OPERATIVE TECHNIQUE (MODIFIED-BRUNELLI TENODESIS)

The authors' preferred operative technique for static, reducible SLIL injury is the MBT TLT because it has been studied extensively is considered the gold standard. The detailed description of this procedure can be found in *Operative Techniques: Hand and Wrist Surgery*, Second Edition.[66]

IMMOBILIZATION AND REHABILITATION

Because of the imprecision and lack of predictability with any type of reconstruction for the SLIL injury, we tend to be conservative in our postoperative therapy. We inform the patient that our goal is painless, albeit mostly poor, motion via a stable reconstruction. The wrist is immobilized in a hand-wrist orthosis for 8 weeks to optimize healing. If K-wires are placed, they are cut short and left under the skin to reduce the risk of pin track infection, which may lead to devastating osteomyelitis in the carpus. K-wires are removed at 6 weeks in the operating room under sedation.

We avoid sending patients to therapists who are unfamiliar with wrist reconstruction procedures. Understandably, hand therapists want to maximize recovery. Therefore, they will stress the reconstructed wrist to match the motion of the other wrist; no reconstruction can withstand the level of stress created during aggressive therapy. Our hand therapists educate and guide patients on a home program, with active wrist exercises gentle enough to avoid wrist pain. Typically, patients understand their limitations and will be judicious in doing moderate exercises and wearing their orthoses for protection if they need to engage in heavier activities.

SUMMARY

Surgery to address SLIL injury remains a challenge, particularly when the ligament is not amenable to primary repair. Although many techniques have been developed and modified, long-term data suggest that there is no superior reconstructive method. New techniques have emerged, such as arthroscopic reconstruction of the dorsal and volar SL ligament, scapholunotriquetral tenodesis, and SLAM. Although early biomechanical and clinical results are promising, long-term data are necessary to confirm the durability of these repairs in maintaining normal wrist anatomic relationships and carpal kinematics.

Early diagnosis and surgical treatment remain the best chances for the treatment of SL pathology; however, if the ligament is not amenable to repair, many reconstructive options are available. The surgeon treating SLIL injuries should be knowledgeable regarding the diagnosis, treatment options, and outcomes of treatment for each stage of injury. Progression to wrist arthritis and need for a salvage operation always should be considered when planning treatment of these challenging injuries.

REFERENCES

1. Lee DH, Dickson KF, Bradley EL. The incidence of wrist interosseous ligament and triangular fibrocartilage articular disc disruptions: a cadaveric study. J Hand Surg Am 2004;29(4):676–84.
2. Berger RA. The ligaments of the wrist. A current overview of anatomy with considerations of their potential functions. Hand Clin 1997;13(1):63–82.
3. Gardner MJ, Crisco JJ, Wolfe SW. Carpal kinematics. Hand Clin 2006;22(4):413–20 [abstract: v].
4. Crisco JJ, Coburn JC, Moore DC, et al. In vivo radiocarpal kinematics and the dart thrower's motion. J Bone Joint Surg Am 2005;87(12):2729–40.
5. Leventhal EL, Moore DC, Akelman E, et al. Carpal and forearm kinematics during a simulated hammering task. J Hand Surg Am 2010;35(7):1097–104.
6. Rainbow MJ, Kamal RN, Leventhal E, et al. In vivo kinematics of the scaphoid, lunate, capitate, and third metacarpal in extreme wrist flexion and extension. J Hand Surg Am 2013;38(2):278–88.
7. Kauer JM. The mechanism of the carpal joint. Clin Orthop Relat Res 1986;(202):16–26.
8. Ishikawa J, Cooney WP 3rd, Niebur G, et al. The effects of wrist distraction on carpal kinematics. J Hand Surg Am 1999;24(1):113–20.
9. Bourne MH, Linscheid RL, Dobyns JH. Concomitant scapholunate dissociation and Kienbock's disease. J Hand Surg Am 1991;16(3):460–4.
10. Chang IY, Mutnal A, Evans PJ, et al. Kienbock's disease and scapholunate advanced collapse. Orthopedics 2014;37(9):578–639.
11. Desmarais J, Soong M. Kienbock's disease and scapholunate dissociation after acute wrist trauma. Hand (N Y) 2013;8(1):82–5.
12. Muramatsu K, Ihara K, Tanaka H, et al. Carpal instability in rheumatoid wrists. Rheumatol Int 2004;24(1):34–6.
13. Stabler A, Baumeister RG, Berger H. Carpal instability and secondary degenerative changes in lesions of the radio-carpal ligaments with various etiology. Handchir Mikrochir Plast Chir 1990;22(6):289–95 [in German].
14. Geissler WB. Arthroscopic management of scapholunate instability. J Wrist Surg 2013;2(2):129–35.
15. Lee SK, Desai H, Silver B, et al. Comparison of radiographic stress views for scapholunate dynamic instability in a cadaver model. J Hand Surg Am 2011;36(7):1149–57.

16. Rhee PC, Moran SL, Shin AY. Association between lunate morphology and carpal collapse in cases of scapholunate dissociation. J Hand Surg Am 2009; 34(9):1633–9.

17. Rohman EM, Agel J, Putnam MD, et al. Scapholunate interosseous ligament injuries: a retrospective review of treatment and outcomes in 82 wrists. J Hand Surg Am 2014;39(10):2020–6.

18. Whipple TL. The role of arthroscopy in the treatment of wrist injuries in the athlete. Clin Sports Med 1998; 17(3):623–34.

19. Whipple TL. The role of arthroscopy in the treatment of wrist injuries in the athlete. Clin Sports Med 1992; 11(1):227–38.

20. Darlis NA, Weiser RW, Sotereanos DG. Partial scapholunate ligament injuries treated with arthroscopic debridement and thermal shrinkage. J Hand Surg Am 2005;30(5):908–14.

21. Darlis NA, Kaufmann RA, Giannoulis F, et al. Arthroscopic debridement and closed pinning for chronic dynamic scapholunate instability. J Hand Surg Am 2006;31(3):418–24.

22. Whipple TL. The role of arthroscopy in the treatment of scapholunate instability. Hand Clin 1995;11(1): 37–40.

23. Linscheid RL, Dobyns JH. Treatment of scapholunate dissociation. Rotatory subluxation of the scaphoid. Hand Clin 1992;8(4):645–52.

24. Walsh JJ, Berger RA, Cooney WP. Current status of scapholunate interosseous ligament injuries. J Am Acad Orthop Surg 2002;10(1):32–42.

25. Berger RA. A method of defining palpable landmarks for the ligament-splitting dorsal wrist capsulotomy. J Hand Surg Am 2007;32(8):1291–5.

26. Cohen MS, Taleisnik J. Direct ligamentous repair of scapholunate dissociation with capsulodesis augmentation. Tech Hand Up Extrem Surg 1998;2(1):18–24.

27. Luchetti R, Zorli IP, Atzei A, et al. Dorsal intercarpal ligament capsulodesis for predynamic and dynamic scapholunate instability. J Hand Surg Eur Vol 2010; 35(1):32–7.

28. Szabo RM, Slater RR Jr, Palumbo CF, et al. Dorsal intercarpal ligament capsulodesis for chronic, static scapholunate dissociation: clinical results. J Hand Surg Am 2002;27(6):978–84.

29. Malone, Polatsch CP, Flink DB, et al. Hand Clin 2012;28(3):253–60.

30. Gajendran VK, Peterson B, Slater RR Jr, et al. Long-term outcomes of dorsal intercarpal ligament capsulodesis for chronic scapholunate dissociation. J Hand Surg Am 2007;32(9):1323–33.

31. Pomerance J. Outcome after repair of the scapholunate interosseous ligament and dorsal capsulodesis for dynamic scapholunate instability due to trauma. J Hand Surg Am 2006;31(8):1380–6.

32. Schweizer A, Steiger R. Long-term results after repair and augmentation ligamentoplasty of rotatory subluxation of the scaphoid. J Hand Surg Am 2002; 27(4):674–84.

33. Wyrick JD, Youse BD, Kiefhaber TR. Scapholunate ligament repair and capsulodesis for the treatment of static scapholunate dissociation. J Hand Surg Br 1998;23(6):776–80.

34. Fox JA, Nedeff DD, Bach BR Jr, et al. Anterior cruciate ligament reconstruction with patellar autograft tendon. Clin Orthop Relat Res 2002;(402):53–63.

35. Svoboda SJ, Eglseder WA Jr, Belkoff SM. Autografts from the foot for reconstruction of the scapholunate interosseous ligament. J Hand Surg Am 1995; 20(6):980–5.

36. Davis CA, Culp RW, Hume EL, et al. Reconstruction of the scapholunate ligament in a cadaver model using a bone-ligament-bone autograft from the foot. J Hand Surg Am 1998;23(5):884–92.

37. Cuenod P, Charriere E, Papaloizos MY. A mechanical comparison of bone-ligament-bone autografts from the wrist for replacement of the scapholunate ligament. J Hand Surg Am 2002;27(6): 985–90.

38. Harvey EJ, Berger RA, Osterman AL, et al. Bone-tissue-bone repairs for scapholunate dissociation. J Hand Surg Am 2007;32(2):256–64.

39. Weiss AP. Scapholunate ligament reconstruction using a bone-retinaculum-bone autograft. J Hand Surg Am 1998;23(2):205–15.

40. Shin SS, Moore DC, McGovern RD, et al. Scapholunate ligament reconstruction using a bone-retinaculum-bone autograft: a biomechanic and histologic study. J Hand Surg Am 1998;23(2):216–21.

41. Wolf JM, Weiss AP. Bone-retinaculum-bone reconstruction of scapholunate ligament injuries. Orthop Clin North Am 2001;32(2):241–6, viii.

42. Soong M, Merrell GA, Ortmann F 4th, et al. Long-term results of bone-retinaculum-bone autograft for scapholunate instability. J Hand Surg Am 2013; 38(3):504–8.

43. Werther JR, Guelmi K, Mazodier F, et al. Use of the extensor retinaculum as a donor site for bone-ligament-bone grafts. Surg Radiol Anat 2001;23(5): 295–9.

44. Harvey EJ, Hanel D, Knight JB, et al. Autograft replacements for the scapholunate ligament: a biomechanical comparison of hand-based autografts. J Hand Surg Am 1999;24(5):963–7.

45. Harvey EJ, Sen M, Martineau P. A vascularized technique for bone-tissue-bone repair in scapholunate dissociation. Tech Hand Up Extrem Surg 2006; 10(3):166–72.

46. Blatt G. Capsulodesis in reconstructive hand surgery. Dorsal capsulodesis for the unstable scaphoid and volar capsulodesis following excision of the distal ulna. Hand Clin 1987;3(1):81–102.

47. Moran SL, Ford KS, Wulf CA, et al. Outcomes of dorsal capsulodesis and tenodesis for treatment of

scapholunate instability. J Hand Surg Am 2006;
31(9):1438–46.

48. Rosenwasser MP, Miyasajsa KC, Strauch RJ. The
RASL procedure: reduction and association of the
scaphoid and lunate using the Herbert screw. Tech
Hand Up Extrem Surg 1997;1(4):263–72.

49. Caloia M, Caloia H, Pereira E. Arthroscopic scapholunate joint reduction. Is an effective treatment for
irreparable scapholunate ligament tears? Clin Orthop Relat Res 2012;470(4):972–8.

50. Aviles AJ, Lee SK, Hausman MR. Arthroscopic
reduction-association of the scapholunate. Arthroscopy 2007;23(1):105.e1–5.

51. Cognet JM, Levadoux M, Martinache X. The use of
screws in the treatment of scapholunate instability.
J Hand Surg Eur Vol 2011;36(8):690–3.

52. Larson TB, Stern PJ. Reduction and association of
the scaphoid and lunate procedure: short-term clinical and radiographic outcomes. J Hand Surg Am
2014;39(11):2168–74.

53. Vitale MA, Shin AY. Avascular necrosis of the
scaphoid following a scapholunate screw: a case
report. Hand (N Y) 2013;8(1):110–4.

54. Corella F, Del Cerro M, Larrainzar-Garijo R, et al.
Arthroscopic ligamentoplasty (bone-tendon-tenode-
sis). A new surgical technique for scapholunate
instability: preliminary cadaver study. J Hand Surg
Eur Vol 2011;36(8):682–9.

55. Corella F, Del Cerro M, Ocampos M, et al. Arthroscopic ligamentoplasty of the dorsal and volar portions of the scapholunate ligament. J Hand Surg
Am 2013;38(12):2466–77.

56. Brunelli GA, Brunelli GR. A new technique to correct
carpal instability with scaphoid rotary subluxation: a
preliminary report. J Hand Surg Am 1995;20(3 Pt 2):
S82–5.

57. Van Den Abbeele KL, Loh YC, Stanley JK, et al.
Early results of a modified Brunelli procedure for
scapholunate instability. J Hand Surg Br 1998;
23(2):258–61.

58. Garcia-Elias M, Lluch AL, Stanley JK. Three-liga-
ment tenodesis for the treatment of scapholunate
dissociation: indications and surgical technique.
J Hand Surg Am 2006;31(1):125–34.

59. Bain GI, Watts AC, McLean J, et al. Cable-
augmented, quad ligament tenodesis scapholunate
reconstruction: rationale, surgical technique, and
preliminary results. Tech Hand Up Extrem Surg
2013;17(1):13–9.

60. Kalb K, Blank S, van Schoonhoven J, et al. Stabilization of the scaphoid according to Brunelli as modified by Garcia-Elias, Lluch, and Stanley for the
treatment of chronic scapholunate dissociation.
Oper Orthop Traumatol 2009;21(4–5):429–41 [in
German].

61. Chabas JF, Gay A, Valenti D, et al. Results of the
modified Brunelli tenodesis for treatment of scapholunate instability: a retrospective study of 19 patients. J Hand Surg Am 2008;33(9):1469–77.

62. Nienstedt F. Treatment of static scapholunate instability with modified Brunelli tenodesis: results over
10 years. J Hand Surg Am 2013;38(5):887–92.

63. Ross M, Loveridge J, Cutbush K, et al. Scapholunate ligament reconstruction. J Wrist Surg 2013;
2(2):110–5.

64. Hsu JW, Kollitz KM, Jegapragasan M, et al. Radiographic evaluation of the modified Brunelli technique versus a scapholunotriquetral transosseous
tenodesis technique for scapholunate dissociation.
J Hand Surg Am 2014;39(6):1041–9.

65. Lee SK, Zlotolow DA, Sapienza A, et al. Biomechanical comparison of 3 methods of scapholunate ligament reconstruction. J Hand Surg Am 2014;39(4):
643–50.

66. Chung KC. Operative techniques: hand and wrist
surgery. 2nd edition. Philadelphia: Elsevier Saunders; 2012.

Bone-Retinaculum-Bone Autografts for Scapholunate Interosseous Ligament Reconstruction

Nathan T. Morrell, MD, Arnold-Peter C. Weiss, MD*

KEYWORDS

- Scapholunate instability • Autograft • Ligament reconstruction

KEY POINTS

- A reducible scapholunate (SL) gap is necessary in order to use a bone-retinaculum-bone (BRB) autograft for scapholunate reconstruction.
- Reduce the SL gap and correct the dorsal intercalated segment instability deformity with Kirschner wires before graft placement.
- Carefully remove a small gap (2–3 mm) of the bone in the midportion of the autograft block taken from the Lister tubercle to avoid any damage to the periosteal/retinacular bridge connecting the resulting 2 bone blocks.
- Prepare the 2 troughs in the scaphoid and lunate carefully to fit the blocks of bone from the BRB autograft. If it is necessary to size the graft to fit the troughs, do so carefully with a rongeur.
- Immobilize for 8 weeks in a cast postoperatively.

INTRODUCTION: NATURE OF THE PROBLEM

Carpal instability arising from an injury to the scapholunate interosseous ligament (SLIL) is commonly seen and treated by hand surgeons. Injury to the SLIL allows the scaphoid to flex while the lunate assumes an extended position; this has been termed dorsal intercalated segment instability (DISI). Left untreated, DISI may progress to scapholunate advanced collapse (SLAC), resulting in a predictable sequence of degenerative changes about the wrist.[1] Several surgical interventions have been described in an attempt to improve wrist kinematics and to prevent the development of these degenerative changes. These interventions include, but are not limited to, primary repair of the ligament; capsulodesis; tenodesis; screw fixation; limited arthrodesis; and a variety of ligament reconstruction techniques, including

bone–soft tissue–bone ligament reconstruction.[2–4] There is general dissatisfaction with the outcomes following primary repair of an acute SLIL tear; there is even more controversy regarding the treatment of chronic tears of the SLIL.[2] No technique to this date has proved to provide optimal results. Recently, attention has shifted toward replacement of the dorsal aspect of the SLIL, which is the most structurally and functionally important aspect of the SLIL.[2]

The need for a surgical technique that provides lasting pain relief, normalized wrist kinematics, and decreased incidence of SLAC wrist degenerative changes is evident.[3] Based on the use of bone–patellar tendon–bone autograft for anterior cruciate ligament reconstruction of the knee, Weiss[4] described the use of bone-retinaculum-bone (BRB) autograft for the treatment of SLIL injuries.

Department of Orthopedics, Brown University, 2 Dudley Street, Suite 200, Providence, RI 02905, USA
* Corresponding author.
E-mail address: apcweiss@brown.edu

Hand Clin 31 (2015) 451–456
http://dx.doi.org/10.1016/j.hcl.2015.04.012
0749-0712/15/$ – see front matter © 2015 Elsevier Inc. All rights reserved.

SURGICAL TECHNIQUE
Preoperative Planning

Preoperative history and physical examination are essential. Confirmation of the diagnosis of SLIL tear follows. Posteroanterior and lateral radiographs are also necessary to assess for degenerative changes. Wrist arthroscopy may also be used as a surgical adjunct to verify the diagnosis and quality of tissue present, as well as to assess the condition of the relevant articular cartilage.

Indications for BRB autograft:
- Complete, irreparable SLIL tears (acute or early chronic)
- Dynamic scapholunate (SL) instability or static SL instability with SL gap greater than 4 mm
- Lunate is not translated ulnarly more than 50% off lunate fossa
- SL interval is easily and fully reducible
- Absence of radiocarpal, midcarpal, or intercarpal arthritic changes
- Native Lister tubercle

Contraindications:
- Irreducible SL interval
- Degenerative changes within the radiocarpal, midcarpal, or intercarpal joints
- Ulnar translation of the lunate more than 50% off the lunate fossa
- Disruption of Lister tubercle (eg, previous surgery or fracture)

Prep and Patient Positioning

- Standard surgical prep
- Supine positioning with arm board

Surgical Approach

- Standard dorsal approach to the SL interval
- Tourniquet control

Surgical Procedure (as Described by Weiss[4])

Approach
- A dorsal longitudinal incision of 6 to 8 cm centered over the Lister tubercle is made.
- The subcutaneous tissue is elevated down to the level of the extensor retinaculum. Care is taken to protect small branches of the superficial radial nerve and to achieve hemostasis.
- The third dorsal compartment is incised and the extensor pollicis longus (EPL) tendon is transposed.
- The dorsal wrist capsule is incised longitudinally between the second and fourth dorsal compartments to expose the SL interval. At this juncture the SLIL is inspected; if robust

enough, a primary repair should be performed. If the SLIL is irreparable but the SL interval is reducible, a reconstruction using BRB autograft is performed (**Fig. 1**).

Graft preparation
- The Lister tubercle is identified and an area measuring 20 mm × 8 mm is marked out.
- A bone block, including the overlying retinaculum and periosteum, is harvested using a small osteotome resulting in a 20 mm × 8 mm × 8 mm autograft of bone (cortical and cancellous), periosteum, and adherent retinaculum.
- A fine-tipped rongeur is used to prepare the autograft and remove the central 2 to 3 mm of cortical and cancellous bone perpendicular to the long axis of the graft. It is critical to preserve the overlying retinaculum and periosteum (**Fig. 2**). The BRB autograft is then wrapped in a saline-dampened gauze and set aside until ready for use.

SL interval preparation
- Kirschner wires (1.73 mm [0.068 inch]) are then drilled into the scaphoid and lunate and used as joysticks to reduce the SL interval.
- The SL interval is percutaneously pinned in position using two 1.14- mm (0.045-inch)

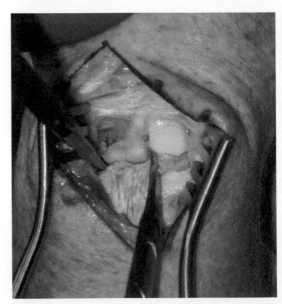

Fig. 1. Using a dorsal exposure to the wrist joint, the scapholunate ligament is examined and the easy of reduction of the scapholunate interval assessed. (*From* Soong M, Merrell GA, Ortmann F 4th, et al. Long-term results of bone-retinaculum-bone autograft for scapholunate instability. J Hand Surg Am 2013;38(3):504–8; with permission.)

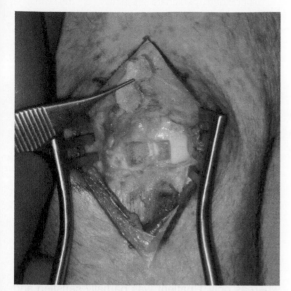

Fig. 2. The BRB autograft is removed from the Lister tubercle vertically and then the midportion of the cancellous and cortical bone is removed using a 2-mm rongeur taking care not to disrupt the periosteum and retinaculum forming the BRB graft (in the forceps). Two troughs are then made in the scaphoid and lunate using a small osteotome and small curette of the size to accept the bone plugs from the BRB graft. (*From* Soong M, Merrell GA, Ortmann F 4th, et al. Long-term results of bone-retinaculum-bone autograft for scapholunate instability. J Hand Surg Am 2013;38(3):504–8; with permission.)

Kirschner wires. These pins must be placed in the volar half of the scaphoid and lunate so as not to interfere with placement of the BRB autograft in the dorsal half of these bones later during the procedure. If necessary, a third wire may be inserted from the scaphoid to the capitate for additional fixation.

- Fluoroscopic images are taken to verify acceptable reduction of the SL joint.
- The recipient sites on the dorsal scaphoid and lunate are prepared with a small osteotome and curette. The trough is shaped such that the bone blocks of the BRB autograft have a snug fit; the BRB autograft may need to be trimmed to accommodate the trough.
- The autograft is then inserted into the prepared troughs with firm manual pressure. The wrist is extended approximately 30°, allowing the dorsal lip of the distal radius to fully seat the bone blocks. Once seated, the BRB autograft should allow full radiocarpal flexion and extension.
- One miniscrew (1.1–1.5 mm in diameter) is used to secure both the scaphoid and lunate bone blocks. The screw is tightened so that the screw head countersinks into the soft

tissue but not through the cortical bone (**Fig. 3**). Fluoroscopy is obtained to confirm Kirschner wire and screw placement (**Fig. 4**).

Closure
- The dorsal capsule is repaired with slight imbrication. If desired, additional reinforcement may be performed using a reverse Blatt capsulodesis.
- The retinaculum is closed with the EPL tendon left transposed above the retinaculum.
- The skin is closed in a method preferred by the surgeon and a sterile dressing applied.
- A short-arm, thumb spica splint (thumb interphalangeal joint free) with the wrist in approximately 20° to 30° of extension is then fabricated.

Immediate Postoperative Care

- Approximately 7 to 10 days postoperatively, the splint is taken down and sutures removed.
- The patient is then placed in a short-arm, thumb spica cast with the wrist in approximately 10° of extension (thumb interphalangeal joint free).
- Following an additional 6 to 7 weeks of cast immobilization, the Kirschner wires placed at the time of surgery are removed.

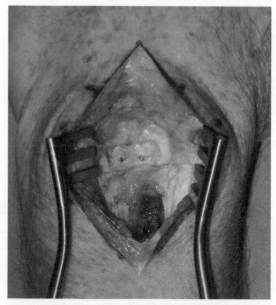

Fig. 3. The BRB graft is then inserted with finger pressure and 1 miniscrew is placed into the scaphoid and another into the lunate, fixing the BRB graft in place. (*From* Soong M, Merrell GA, Ortmann F 4th, et al. Long-term results of bone-retinaculum-bone autograft for scapholunate instability. J Hand Surg Am 2013;38(3):504–8; with permission.)

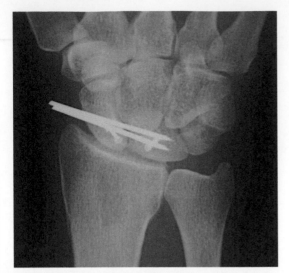

Fig. 4. A radiograph shows the Kirschner wires transfixing the scaphoid and lunate in a reduced fashion as well as the 2 miniscrews maintaining BRB placement.

REHABILITATION AND RECOVERY

Supervised hand therapy is commenced at approximately 8 weeks postoperatively (ie, following Kirschner wire removal). This therapy consists of gentle active and passive range-of-motion exercises with the goal of slowly increasing wrist range of motion. Patients should be educated that forceful active motion may risk injury to the graft for 3 to 4 months postoperatively. Strengthening exercises begin at approximately 12 weeks postoperatively.

CLINICAL RESULTS IN THE LITERATURE

The initial clinical series of this technique presented an average follow-up of 3.6 years (range, 24–54 months) for 19 patients.[4] The results were separated based on whether the preoperative scapholunate instability was dynamic or static; typically patients with dynamic instability fared better with the procedure. In general, wrist flexion and extension decreased from preoperative values, whereas grip strength improved and patients were satisfied. Minor complications occurred in 32% of patients; most commonly neuropraxia of the sensory branch of the radial nerve. No infections, donor site discomfort, or extensor adhesions were noted.

Dynamic Instability

Of the 14 patients with dynamic instability who underwent the procedure, 12 had no pain postoperatively and 2 had pain only with wrist activity. Thirteen of the 14 patients were completely satisfied and returned to their previous work activities, whereas only 1 patient was partially satisfied and required modified work activities. Postoperative wrist flexion averaged 67° and extension averaged 52°, compared with preoperative 72° and 69°, respectively. Average grip strength improved from 26.8 kg (59 lb) to 39.0 kg (86 lb). Postoperative radiographs showed an average SL angle of 50° and an SL gap of less than or equal to 3 mm in 13 patients. One patient had a gap of 4 mm on the power grip view but was asymptomatic.

Static Instability

Of the 5 patients with static instability who underwent the procedure, 2 had no pain, 1 had pain only with activity, and 2 continued to experience constant pain postoperatively. One patient was completely satisfied, 2 were partially satisfied, and 2 were dissatisfied; 3 underwent additional salvage procedures because of continued pain. Postoperative wrist flexion averaged 42° and

Table 1
Summary of early and long-term results

	Preoperative (N = 14)	Early (N = 14)	Long-term (n = 9)
Follow-up (y)	—	3.6	11.9
Failures	—	0	3
SL Angle (°)	<60	50	60
SL Gap (mm)	2	<3	3.5
Arthritis Grade	0	0	1
Wrist Extension (°)	69	52	44
Wrist Flexion (°)	72	67	53
Grip Strength (kg)	26.8	39.0	35.8
Mayo Score	65	87	83

From Soong M, Merrell GA, Ortmann F 4th, et al. Long-term results of bone-retinaculum-bone autograft for scapholunate instability. J Hand Surg Am 2013;38(3):506; with permission.

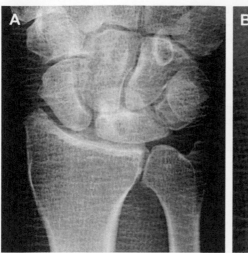
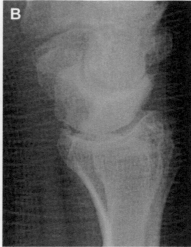

Fig. 5. A 15-year follow-up on a patient with a BRB autograft without miniscrew fixation shows secondary mild to moderate midcarpal arthritic changes but a well-aligned SL gap on the posteroanterior radiograph (*A*) and a fairly well-aligned lunate on the lateral radiograph (*B*). The patient had no pain with activity.

extension averaged 44°, compared with preoperative 68° and 64°, respectively. Average grip strength improved from 16.8 kg (37 lb) to 21.8 kg (48 lb). Postoperative radiographs showed an average SL angle of 64° and an SL gap of less than or equal to 3 mm in only 2 patients.

Longer term results have been reported on most of the initial cohort of patients with dynamic scapholunate instability (**Table 1**).[5] In general, clinical and radiographic outcomes deteriorated moderately from the prior report. Three patients (21%) required a salvage procedure between 2 and 4 years following the index procedure. At the time of reoperation in these patients, 1 of the BRB grafts remained intact, 1 was partially torn, and 1 was completely resorbed. Six of the initial patients (43%) were available for long-term clinical evaluation. For these patients, follow-up averaged 11.9 years (range, 10.7–14.1 years). At final follow-up, wrist flexion averaged 53° and extension averaged 44°; an overall decrease of 22° in the flexion-extension arc from the short-term results. Average grip strength decreased slightly from 39.0 kg (86 lb) to 35.8 kg (79 lb). The average scapholunate angle increased from 50° to 65° and the SL gap averaged 3.5 mm (range, 2–10 mm). Wrist arthritis progressed to an average of SLAC stage I (**Fig. 5**).

Although the clinical and radiographic results seem to deteriorate in the long term, similar to other soft tissue reconstructive techniques, the BRB technique did prove durable in some patients. The strength and stiffness of the BRB graft has been questioned. In a cadaveric study, Shin and colleagues[3] found that the BRB autograft

was significant weaker than the dorsal SLIL. This weakness seemed to be caused by a 3-fold difference in size because the failure stress (failure force per cross-sectional area) was not significantly different between the two tissues. Nevertheless, it seems that bone–soft tissue–bone autografts are an important treatment option for SLIL reconstruction; more research is needed to identify the ideal graft with long-term durability.

SUMMARY

Carpal instability arising from an injury to the SLIL may lead to a predictable pattern of degenerative changes about the wrist (ie, SLAC wrist). There is a demand for a surgical technique that provides lasting pain relief, normalized wrist kinematics, and decreased development of SLAC wrist. Recently, attention has shifted toward replacement of the dorsal aspect of the SLIL. Based on the use of bone–patellar tendon–bone autograft for anterior cruciate ligament reconstruction of the knee, Weiss[4] described the use of BRB autograft for the treatment of SLIL injuries. This technique uses bone from the distal radius with periosteum and extensor retinaculum bridging between 2 bone blocks. The graft is readily available with minimal morbidity. SLIL reconstruction with the BRB autograft results in satisfactory outcomes in the short term, especially in patients with dynamic rather than static SL instability. However, like other soft tissue SLIL reconstruction techniques, the long-term durability of the BRB technique is variable. More research is needed to determine the ideal tissue source, although it seems that a bone–soft tissue–bone reconstructive technique is a good option and will be a part of the hand surgeon's armamentarium in the future.

REFERENCES

1. Watson HK, Ballet FL. The SLAC wrist: scapholunate advanced collapse pattern of degenerative arthritis. J Hand Surg Am 1984;9(3):358–65.
2. Harvey EJ, Berger RA, Osterman AL, et al. Bone-tissue-bone repairs for scapholunate dissociation. J Hand Surg Am 2007;32(2):256–64.
3. Shin SS, Moore DC, McGovern RD, et al. Scapholunate ligament reconstruction using a bone-retinaculum-bone autograft: a biomechanic and histologic study. J Hand Surg Am 1998;23(2):216–21.
4. Weiss AP. Scapholunate ligament reconstruction using a bone-retinaculum-bone autograft. J Hand Surg Am 1998;23(2):205–15.
5. Soong M, Merrell GA, Ortmann F 4th, et al. Long-term results of bone-retinaculum-bone autograft for scapholunate instability. J Hand Surg Am 2013;38(3):504–8.

Chronic Scapholunate Ligament Injuries
Treatment with Supplemental Fixation

Jason W. Dahl, MD, Jerry I. Huang, MD*

KEYWORDS

- Scapholunate instability • RASL • SLAM • Reconstruction

KEY POINTS

- Several techniques for supplemental fixation have been described for scapholunate (SL) ligament reconstruction to address concerns of recurrent SL diastasis with other reconstructive procedures.
- Screw fixation with use of RASL (reduction and association of the scaphoid and lunate) screws may allow compression and more rigid fixation.
- There are limited clinical series of outcomes of temporary or permanent screw fixation for SL reconstruction.
- The SL axis method (SLAM) technique places a tendon graft across the SL axis in addition to dorsal reconstruction to allow a stronger construct compared with the modified Brunelli technique.
- For both the RASL and SLAM techniques, it is critical to place SL fixation along the isometric axis of the SL joint to minimize risk of iatrogenic fracture of the scaphoid or lunate and congruent joint reduction.

INTRODUCTION

The management of chronic scapholunate (SL) ligament injuries remains a difficult problem for the treating hand surgeon. Untreated SL dissociation leads to progressive carpal collapse and the development of SL advanced collapse (SLAC) with degeneration of the radiocarpal and midcarpal joints. There is usually inadequate ligament remaining for direct repair in injuries older than 6 to 8 weeks. Despite decades of research and the development of numerous surgical techniques, no single procedure has come forward as being superior in restoring carpal kinematics and maintaining reduction over time. Because of the unpredictable outcomes from chronic SL reconstruction, with a large number of patients developing SL gapping and development of arthritic changes on radiographs, some investigators have advocated limited intercarpal fusion for primary treatment of chronic SL ligament injuries.[1–3]

With most of the described dorsal capsulodeses, the procedure reduces the SL angle but does not directly correct the diastasis. In a series of patients undergoing either Blatt or Mayo dorsal capsulodesis, Moran and colleagues[4] found progressive radiographic deterioration at a mean follow-up of 54 months, with increase in the SL gap from 2.7 to 3.9 mm. Similar progressive diastasis was shown by Pomerance,[5] with an increase in SL gap of 6 mm in high-demand patients with strenuous jobs. The modified Brunelli technique (MBT) is superior biomechanically in maintaining SL angle and preventing SL diastasis with physiologic loading.[6] However, Moran and colleagues[7] found similar improvement in SL angle but progressive SL widening at mean follow-up of 36 months in his series of 15 patients with MBT reconstruction.

In order to improve the reduction and stability of the reconstruction, Ross and colleagues[8] described the scapholunatotriquetral (SLT) tenodesis technique, in which ligament reconstruction

Department of Orthopaedics and Sports Medicine, University of Washington Medical Center, 1959 NE Pacific Street, Seattle, WA 98195, USA
* Corresponding author. 4245 Roosevelt Way Northeast, Box 354740, Seattle, WA 98105.
E-mail address: jihuang@uw.edu

Hand Clin 31 (2015) 457–465
http://dx.doi.org/10.1016/j.hcl.2015.04.003

along the central axis of the SL joint is performed with a tendon graft, in addition to dorsal scapholunate interosseous ligament (SLIL) reconstruction. The SL axis method (SLAM) uses a commercial tendon graft anchor placed into the lunate to perform the central SL stabilization and a tenodesis screw in the scaphoid.

Most SL reconstruction techniques include K-wire fixation across the SL and, sometimes, scaphocapitate joints. However, with pin fixation, there are concerns of inadequate stability of fixation, pin loosening with migration, and pin tract infection. Screw fixation has the advantage of more stable fixation, compression across the SL joint, decreased risk of pin tract infection, and ability to maintain the fixation for a longer period.

This article reviews surgical techniques and the available published literature on supplemental fixation in treatment of chronic SL instability, focusing on open and arthroscopic screw fixation and soft tissue stabilization using the SLAM technique.

PREOPERATIVE PLANNING

Accurate diagnosis of the chronic, static SL injury remains critical when considering the treatment algorithm and supplemental fixation. Acute SL ligament injuries (considered <6 weeks old) can most often be repaired primarily combined with K-wire fixation. In subacute injuries, consideration should be given to high-resolution 3-T MRI to assess the quality of the dorsal SLIL before embarking on surgical repair or reconstruction.

Preoperative radiographs should be obtained and carefully examined for the presence of radiographic changes consistent with arthritis. Radioscaphoid arthritis limited to the radial styloid (stage 1 SLAC) is not a contraindication to the SL reconstruction. This condition is addressed with a simultaneously performed radial styloidectomy to allow better positioning of the screw and tendon reconstruction, as well as to improve radial deviation postoperatively.

Radiographic Imaging

- Neutral posteroanterior (PA), lateral, and oblique views
- PA views in radial and ulnar deviation
- Bilateral pencil-grip PA views
- Comparison films of the contralateral wrist

Indications

- Chronic, static SL instability with widening and dorsal intercalated segment instability deformity that is easily reducible intraoperatively
- Irreparable acute SL injuries
- Chronic SL instability with limited, focal arthritic changes over the radial styloid (stage 1 SLAC)
- Salvage after failed previous ligament repair or reconstruction

Contraindications

- Static SL instability that is not easily reducible
- Advanced radioscaphoid, capitolunate, or arthritic changes

SURGICAL APPROACH

We use a standard open dorsal approach to the wrist with a ligament-sparing dorsal capsulotomy as described by Berger and coleagues.[9] Alternatively, distally based U-shaped capsular flap and T-shaped capsulotomy have been described.

Once the SL interval is identified, close inspection of the articular integrity of the radiocarpal and midcarpal joints should be undertaken. Degenerative changes involving the distal pole of the scaphoid and tip of the radial styloid can be managed with a radial styloidectomy. Patients with extensive radioscaphoid or capitolunate joint degenerative arthritis should be managed with a proximal row carpectomy or limited intercarpal fusion.

SCREW FIXATION OF THE SCAPHOLUNATE JOINT

The use of screw fixation was first described by Rosenwasser and colleagues[10] in the reduction and association of the scaphoid and lunate (RASL) procedure in a 1997 technique article. To address static, irreparable SL instability, an open reassociation of the SL interval using a permanent headless screw was proposed. The key to this procedure is the dechondrification of the SL articulating surfaces to create a fibrous nonunion to maintain long-term reduction and stability. More recently, others have described arthroscopic RASL (ARASL) as a minimally invasive alternative to the open procedure. Larson and colleagues used a temporary screw to augment the soft tissue reconstruction that is removed at 4 months postoperatively.

For screw placement, a second radial column incision is made directly over the first dorsal compartment, starting just proximal to the radial styloid. Branches of the radial sensory nerve are identified, mobilized, and protected. The extensor retinaculum is incised longitudinally with release of the first dorsal compartment. A longitudinal incision is made in the capsule allowing access to the scaphoid waist and radial styloid.

A limited radial styloidectomy may be performed using an osteotome or saw. The styloidectomy addresses any arthritic changes present while providing access for proper headless screw placement in the scaphoid. Care is taken to limit the resection size to 3 to 4 mm to maintain the origin of the radioscaphocapitate ligament and decrease the risk for radiocarpal instability that may result from over-resection.[11]

In addition to SL diastasis, there is rotatory subluxation of the scaphoid and lunate. Reduction is achieved with the use of 1.4-mm (0.054-inch) K-wires as joysticks placed into the scaphoid and lunate. The first K-wire is placed over the distal-radial aspect of the flexed scaphoid and aimed proximally, whereas the second lunate K-wire is placed over the ulnar aspect of the extended lunate and aimed proximal to distal. To avoid impeding screw placement, the K-wires should not be placed in the center of the carpal bones. In the RASL procedure, the SL interval is opened and the articular surfaces are debrided through the articular cartilage and subchondral bone using a rongeur and 3-mm surgical burr down to cancellous bleeding surface. Care is taken to avoid removing too much bone because that would make it more difficult to close the gap.

The K-wires are brought together to reduce the diastasis as well as to extend the scaphoid and flex the lunate. Failure to anatomically reduce extended lunate results in limited wrist extension and abnormal loading of the capitolunate joint, which may lead to hastened degeneration in this articulation. Radiographically, the correction of

the lateral SL angle (approximately 45°–50°), restoration of the Gilula arc, and colinearity of the lunate and capitate should be assessed. Once achieved, the reduction is maintained with a clamp across the K-wires or held by an assistant.

A guidewire for a cannulated headless compression screw is placed through the radial column incision starting immediately proximal to the scaphoid waist, aiming toward the center of the SL joint. Ideal placement of the guidewire is centered in the lunate and scaphoid in both planes to establish an isometric rotation point. Commercially available jigs may be used to assist with guidewire placement; however, we prefer using a free-hand technique. Care must be taken not to start too distal in the scaphoid and enter the midcarpal joint. Similarly, a starting point too proximal risks iatrogenic fracture through the proximal articular surfaces of the scaphoid or lunate. With placement of a permanent headless RASL screw, we subtract 6 mm from the measurement to ensure subchondral placement and avoid future impingement on the distal radius. If the screw is temporary, then the screw should be left 1 to 2 mm short to facilitate removal at a later time. For temporary screws, a headed or headless screw can be used. Compression of the SL joint is visualized directly. There are several different headless compression screws that may be used. It is important that the central portion that crosses the SL joint is smooth and nonthreaded (**Fig. 1**).

In the RASL procedure as described by Rosenwasser and colleagues,[10] no capsulodesis or any other soft tissue reconstruction is performed. We typically perform a Mayo Clinic dorsal intercarpal (DIC) capsulodesis or MBT combined with

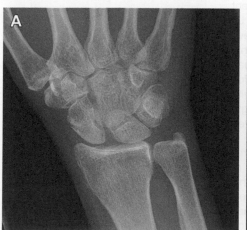
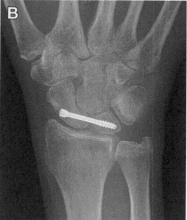

Fig. 1. Preoperative radiograph showing a chronic SL disruption (*A*). Postoperative radiograph showing reduction of the SL interval and placement of a temporary RASL screw after a dorsal capsulodesis (*B*). (*Courtesy of* Jeff Friedrich, MD.)

screw augmentation. The joint capsule is closed, followed by repair of the extensor retinaculum, leaving the extensor pollicis longus tendon externalized.

POSTOPERATIVE CARE AND REHABILITATION

A sterile dressing is placed and a short-arm thumb spica splint is applied. At the first postoperative visit at 2 weeks, repeat radiographs are obtained, and the wrist is placed in a thumb spica cast for another 4 weeks. At 6 weeks, casts are discontinued, the patient is transitioned to a removable splint, and active range-of-motion exercises are begun. Passive range of motion and return to activities of daily living are begun at 12 weeks. We prefer to remove our screws at 6 months and do not leave the screws in permanently. Following screw removal, patients may return to full, unrestricted activities.

CLINICAL RESULTS IN THE LITERATURE

There is a paucity of literature on clinical outcomes of screw fixation in SL ligament reconstruction. Since the initial description in 1997, White and colleagues[12] presented outcomes in a series of 32 patients at an average follow-up of 6 years. Flexion-extension arc was 80% and grip strength 90% of the contralateral side, with a favorable mean DASH (Disabilities of the Arm, Shoulder, and Hand) score of 16.6. Radiographic follow-up showed a significant reduction in SL gap and SL angle versus preoperative radiographs. Treatment failure occurred in only 2 of 32 patients who went on to require salvage procedures for progressive SLAC wrist deformity.

An ARASL procedure was described by Aviles and colleagues[13] with arthroscopic debridement and decortication of the SL joint, followed by placement of a headless compression screw. Caloia and colleagues[14] reported on 8 patients with an arthroscopic RASL procedure with mean follow-up of 34.6 months. Patients had reduction in pain with improvement in function overall, with 80% range of movement and 78% grip strength compared with the contralateral wrist. However, 3 screws were removed because of loosening.

With placement of an SL screw, concerns include screw loosening, iatrogenic scaphoid or lunate fracture, and screw breakage. The original design on the scapholunate intercarpal screw (Acumed, Portland, OR) was discontinued because of such concerns. Cognet and colleagues[15] reported on 7 patients with chronic SL instability treated with ARASL and had a 100% complication rate with partial destruction of the

scaphoid and/or lunate in all 7 cases. Larson and Stern[16] recently reported short-term outcomes in a case series of 7 patients (8 wrists) who underwent an open RASL procedure. There was radiographic failure in 5 out of 8 wrists with progressive loss of SL gap reduction and increase in SL angle (**Fig. 2**). Despite the high rate of radiographic failure, disability in the failed wrists remained low as determined by DASH and patient rated wrist evaluation (PRWE) outcome scores. Based on their findings, the investigators recommended seeking alternative procedures to address chronic SL instability.

In a separate study, Larson and colleagues[17] compared the results of temporary screw fixation with K-wire fixation in SL ligament reconstruction and found an improvement in both the immediate postoperative gap (3.1 vs 1.3 mm) and better maintenance of the SL gap and angle in the screw cohort. The investigators recommend removing the screw at 4 months postoperatively. Based on their experience, this was sufficient time for ligament healing but also the time point at which they observed evidence of screw loosening.

The published literature is sparse and conflicting, offering little guidance to the treating hand surgeon. Until further outcomes evidence is available, surgeons must rely on their own experiences, training, and clinical judgment when addressing

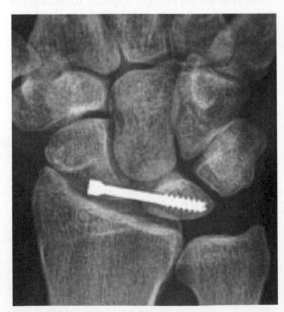

Fig. 2. Radiograph taken 3 months after the RASL procedure shows early signs of screw loosening and migration with loss of coronal plane reduction. (*From* Larson TB, Stern PJ. Reduction and association of the scaphoid and lunate procedure: short-term clinical and radiographic outcomes. J Hand Surg Am 2014;39(11):2171; with permission.)

this difficult problem. We currently decorticate the articular surfaces similar to the RASL technique but routinely remove the screw between 4 and 6 months postoperatively to minimize risk of screw loosening, breakage, or cutout through the carpal bones.

SCAPHOLUNATE AXIS METHOD

The SLAM is a recent addition to the available SL reconstructive options. The SLAM method uses a tendon graft anchor that allows placement of a tendon graft in the central axis of the SL articulation, thereby tethering the 2 carpal bones together. The remaining tail of the graft exits from the radial side of the scaphoid waist and is placed dorsally across the SL interval, reconstructing the dorsal SLIL. The central placement of the ligament reconstruction provides a more uniform apposition at the SL joint than isolated dorsal reconstructions, which may lead to gapping on the volar aspect. Using a biologic repair for the central-axis fixation may more closely approximate the multiplanar motion seen in the native SL joint and avoid complications such as screw failure that can occur in the RASL procedure.

The surgical approach and incisions are similar to those used in the RASL procedure (discussed earlier). The dorsal wrist is approached through a ligament-sparing approach followed by use of joysticks in the scaphoid and lunate to reduce the joint. Similar to the RASL procedure, a second incision is made over the radial styloid. The starting point is found along the ridge between the proximal articular and the central nonarticular surfaces and immediately dorsal to the midlateral line of the scaphoid. Eccentric placement should be avoided. The starting point is directly visualized

to ensure that a 4-mm drill can be passed without breaching the surrounding cortices.

A commercially available aiming guide can be used to assist with accurate wire placement as well as reduction across the SL joint. The distal arm of the aiming guide should be placed onto the proximal ulnar corner of the lunate, and centered on the lateral view. A small incision may need to be made in the dorsal radiocarpal ligament (DRC) to accommodate the aiming arm. Compression through the aiming guide assists in reducing the SL joint. A 1.6-mm guidewire is placed through the aiming guide and across the SL joint (**Fig. 3**A). Fluoroscopic evaluation is critical to ensure accurate placement. Eccentric pin placement is unacceptable and risks fracture of the scaphoid or lunate. A second K-wire is placed through the jig, distal to this, to stabilize the guide during drilling and graft insertion, and to provide supplemental SL fixation.[18]

Using fluoroscopy, a cannulated step drill is placed over the SL guidewire and drilled across the SL joint into the lunate (see **Fig. 3**B). The SL guidewire and drill are removed and the drill holes are thoroughly irrigated to flush any remaining debris. Residual drill debris may impede the smooth passage of the tendon graft.

Autograft tendon is harvested. Palmaris longus is our first choice for graft, but, if absent, one-third of the flexor carpi radialis tendon may be used. We obtain as long a tendon graft as possible, with the goal of a minimum of 12 cm. The tendon graft is whip-stitched on both ends with a suture to tubularize the tendon. The tendon is then threaded through the graft anchor to create a 2-tailed tendon graft (**Fig. 4**).

The tendon graft anchor is next passed through the scaphoid and seated into the lunate. With the tendon tails under tension, a tenodesis screw

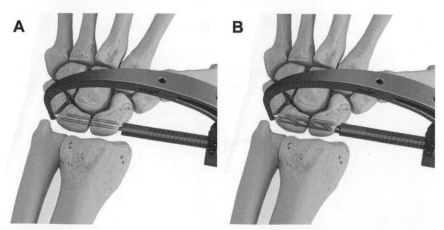

Fig. 3. Use of an aiming guide to reduce the SL interval and center the SL axis guidewire. A second parallel K-wire is placed to maintain the reduction (A). A step drill is next used across the SL joint (B). (*Courtesy of* Arthrex, Inc, Naples, FL; with permission.)

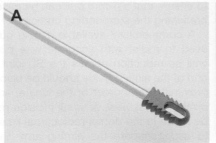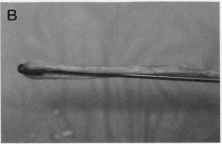

Fig. 4. Palmaris longus autograft is threaded through the anchor (*A*) to create a 2-tailed graft (*B*). (*Courtesy of* Arthrex, Inc, Naples, FL; with permission.)

may be placed into scaphoid to secure the tendon graft (**Fig. 5**A). Screw placement may help reduce the effect of creep on the graft construct; however, we do not routinely use this method. Instead we use the dorsal tendon fixation to provide tension to the graft.

The free ends of the graft are passed beneath the capsule dorsally and across the SL joint to recreate the dorsal SLIL. Multiple fixation sites are available, including the soft tissues of the DRC or lunotriquetral ligaments. We prefer to place a small suture anchor into the dorsal aspect of the lunate. The graft tails are placed under tension, the SL interval reduced using joysticks as needed, and the tails are tied to the suture anchor and the suture remnants are left uncut.

As a final step to further extend the scaphoid and prevent future palmarflexion, a dorsal capsulodesis is performed by suturing a strip of the DIC ligament onto the suture anchor in the lunate (see **Fig. 5**B). In addition to the supplemental SL pin, we sometimes augment our fixation with a scaphocapitate pin to maintain scaphoid extension and prevent capitate proximal migration.

The joint capsule and extensor retinaculum are closed in standard fashion.

Open-hinge Scapholunate Axis Method

Alternatively, the senior author uses a modification to the procedure discussed earlier that allows free-hand guidewire placement and ensures accurate placement of the tendon graft across the center of the articular surface of the scaphoid and lunate. The same dorsal approach is performed as in the SLAM technique. The joysticks in the scaphoid and lunate are used to open the SL interval so that each surface of the joint can be seen en face, which allows the surgeon to accurately place drill holes in the center of the joint under direct visualization.

The scaphoid and lunate drill holes are performed independently. The guidewire is placed centrally into the lunate, aiming toward the midpoint of the proximal ulnar lunate corner (**Fig. 6**A–C). Once placement is confirmed using fluoroscopic imaging, a cannulated step drill is placed over the guidewire used to prepare the

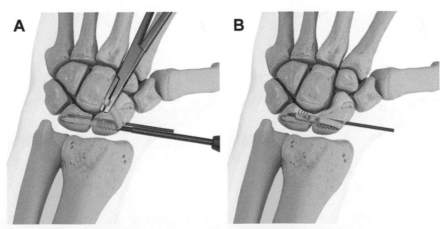

Fig. 5. The graft anchor with the palmaris tendon is inserted across the SL joint and seated in the lunate (*A*). The remnants of the tendon graft are brought around dorsally for reconstruction of the dorsal SL interosseous ligament (*B*). (*Courtesy of* Arthrex, Inc, Naples, FL; with permission.)

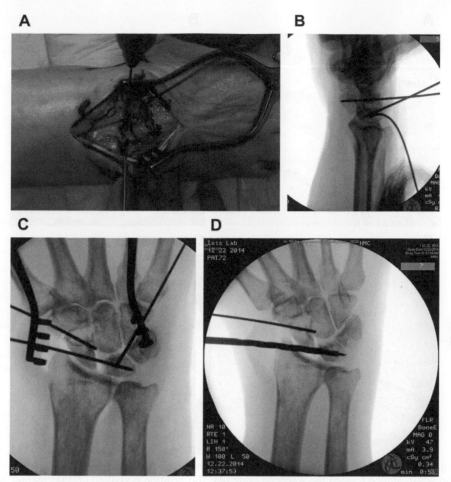

Fig. 6. K-wires in the scaphoid and lunate are used to hinge open the SL interval. The guidewire is placed en face, centrally into the lunate (*A*; dorsal view; left, proximal; right, distal). Fluoroscopic images are obtained to ensure that the guidewire is centered on the PA (*B*) and lateral (*C*) views. With the guidewire in place, the lunate is drilled with the step drill (*D*).

lunate for the graft anchor (see **Fig. 6**D). The guidewire is then placed in the central aspect of the scaphoid and advanced toward the radial side of the scaphoid waist, aiming toward the scaphoid ridge as described previously (**Fig. 7**A, B). Once central placement is confirmed visually and fluoroscopically, the guidewire is advanced through the radial cortex and retrieved through the styloid incision. The scaphoid is then drilled in a radial to ulnar direction using the cannulated step drill (see **Fig. 7**C, D; **Fig. 8**).

Under direct visualization, the tendon anchor is driven into the predrilled hole in the lunate using a mallet. A suture passer is used to draw the free tails of the tendon graft in an ulnar to radial direction through the scaphoid. The tendon graft is then passed dorsally across the SL joint as in the traditional SLAM technique to reconstruct the dorsal SLIL.

Postoperative Care, Rehabilitation, and Recovery

At 2 weeks, repeat radiographs are obtained and skin sutures are removed. The patient is moved into a thumb spica cast for 4 more weeks. At the 6-week visit, we remove the K-wires and transition to a removable thumb spica splint made by our hand therapists. Gentle active and active-assisted range-of-motion exercises are initiated under the guidance of a hand therapist. Passive range of motion and strengthening begin at 12 weeks. Contact sports and activities with a high fall risk are restricted until a full 6 months postoperatively.

CLINICAL RESULTS IN THE LITERATURE

The biomechanical properties of the SLAM technique have been studied in a cadaveric study

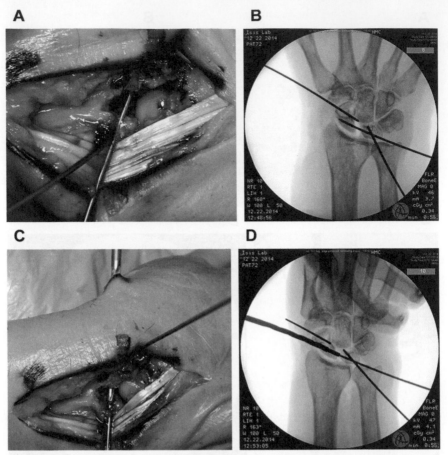

Fig. 7. The guidewire is then placed in the central aspect of the scaphoid and advanced toward the radial side of the scaphoid waist, aiming toward the scaphoid ridge (*A*). This position is verified on fluoroscopic imaging (*B*). The scaphoid is then drilled in a radial to ulnar direction using the cannulated step drill (*C, D*).

comparing the SLAM with 2 other common SL reconstructions: the Blatt capsulodesis and the MBT. The SLAM and MBT were significantly better at maintaining the SL interval compared with the Blatt capsulodesis. The absolute correction in SL angle was highest in the SLAM method, but not statistically different from the other methods. The multiplanar tether of the SL joint with the central

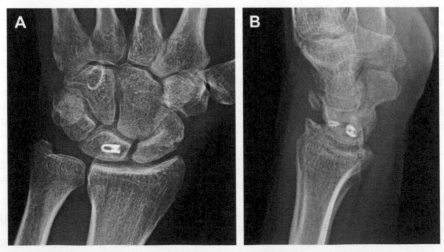

Fig. 8. Final PA (*A*) and lateral (*B*) radiographs 6 months after the SLAM procedure.

reconstruction as well as dorsal reconstruction may help prevent SL gapping and rotatory subluxation better than traditional dorsal-only reconstructions. The dual reconstruction may also reduce tendon creep, which frequently leads to progressive diastasis over time with other tenodesis techniques.

There are no reported clinical outcomes on the SLAM technique currently. Ross and colleagues[8] described the SLT tenodesis technique, which provides a similar central biologic tether and dorsal ligament reconstruction. The investigators have performed this technique on more than 40 patients and reported on the outcomes in 11 patients with more than 12 months of follow-up. Patients had good reduction in pain and improvement in strength and function as assessed by DASH and PRWE questionnaires. The SL gap decreased from 4.2 mm preoperatively to 1.6 mm at the time of follow-up.

SUMMARY

Treatment of chronic SL ligament injuries remains a clinical challenge for hand surgeons. Traditional reconstructive techniques with dorsal capsulodesis and various tenodesis procedures are often disappointing and unpredictable, with frequent loss of reduction with progressive radiographic deterioration with diastasis and degenerative arthritis. Supplemental fixation with use of screws or a tendon graft anchor provide for central reconstruction may allow more robust stabilization of the SL reconstruction. However, there are currently very few clinical data showing superiority of these newer techniques to other soft tissue reconstructions. With screw fixation, there continue to be concerns of complications, including screw loosening and fracture of the scaphoid and/or lunate over time.

REFERENCES

1. Gajendran VK, Peterson B, Slater RR Jr, et al. Long-term outcomes of dorsal intercarpal ligament capsulodesis for chronic scapholunate dissociation. J Hand Surg Am 2007;32(9):1323–33.

2. Kleinman WB, Carroll C 4th. Scapho-trapezio-trapezoid arthrodesis for treatment of chronic static and dynamic scapho-lunate instability: a 10-year perspective on pitfalls and complications. J Hand Surg Am 1990;15(3):408–14.

3. Hastings DE, Silver RL. Intercarpal arthrodesis in the management of chronic carpal instability after trauma. J Hand Surg Am 1984;9(6):834–40.

4. Moran SL, Cooney WP, Berger RA, et al. Capsulodesis for the treatment of chronic scapholunate instability. J Hand Surg Am 2005;30(1):16–23.

5. Pomerance J. Outcome after repair of the scapholunate interosseous ligament and dorsal capsulodesis for dynamic scapholunate instability due to trauma. J Hand Surg Am 2006;31(8):1380–6.

6. Pollock PJ, Sieg RN, Baechler MF, et al. Radiographic evaluation of the modified Brunelli technique versus the Blatt capsulodesis for scapholunate dissociation in a cadaver model. J Hand Surg Am 2010;35(10):1589–98.

7. Moran SL, Ford KS, Wulf CA, et al. Outcomes of dorsal capsulodesis and tenodesis for treatment of scapholunate instability. J Hand Surg Am 2006;31(9):1438–46.

8. Ross M, Loveridge J, Cutbush K, et al. Scapholunate ligament reconstruction. J Wrist Surg 2013;2(2):110–5.

9. Berger RA, Bishop AT, Bettinger PC. New dorsal capsulotomy for the surgical exposure of the wrist. Ann Plast Surg 1995;35(1):54–9.

10. Rosenwasser MP, Miyasaki KC, Strauch RJ. The RASL procedure: reduction and association of the scaphoid and lunate using the Herbert screw. Tech Hand Up Extrem Surg 1997;1(4):263–72.

11. Nakamura T, Cooney WP 3rd, Lui WH, et al. Radial styloidectomy: a biomechanical study on stability of the wrist joint. J Hand Surg Am 2001;26(1):85–93.

12. White NJ, Raskolnikov D, Swart E, et al. Reduction and association of the scaphoid and lunate (RASL): long-term follow-up of a reconstruction technique for chronic scapholunate dissociation. J Bone Joint Surg Br 2012;94(Suppl):51, XXXVIII.

13. Aviles AJ, Lee SK, Hausman MR. Arthroscopic reduction-association of the scapholunate. Arthroscopy 2007;23(1):105.e1–5.

14. Caloia M, Caloia H, Pereira E. Arthroscopic scapholunate joint reduction. Is an effective treatment for irreparable scapholunate ligament tears? Clin Orthop Relat Res 2012;470(4):972–8.

15. Cognet JM, Levadoux M, Martinache X. The use of screws in the treatment of scapholunate instability. J Hand Surg Eur Vol 2011;36(8):690–3.

16. Larson TB, Stern PJ. Reduction and association of the scaphoid and lunate procedure: short-term clinical and radiographic outcomes. J Hand Surg Am 2014;39(11):2168–74.

17. Larson TB, Gaston RG, Chadderdon RC. The use of temporary screw augmentation for the treatment of scapholunate injuries. Tech Hand Up Extrem Surg 2012;16(3):135–40.

18. Lee SK, Zlotolow DA, Sapienza A, et al. Biomechanical comparison of 3 methods of scapholunate ligament reconstruction. J Hand Surg Am 2014;39(4):643–50.

Diagnosis and Treatment of Acute Lunotriquetral Ligament Injuries

 CrossMark

Michael C. Nicoson, MD[a], Steven L. Moran, MD[b],*

KEYWORDS

• Wrist • Ligament • Lunotriquetral • Intercarpal • Arthroscopy

KEY POINTS

• Lunotriquetral (LT) injuries are uncommon entities that require precise clinical evaluation with findings of point tenderness at or surrounding the LT interval.
• Radiographs show typically normal findings in cases of LT ligament injury.
• Diagnostic arthroscopy provides the most accurate means of accessing the LT joint.
• Treatment options for acute LT injury include immobilization, arthroscopic debridement, and direct open repair.

INTRODUCTION

Isolated lunotriquetral interosseous ligament (LTIL) injury is an uncommon and often missed diagnosis. The acute injury typically presents with normal findings on radiographs, and the physical findings can be confounded by other concomitant injuries on the ulnar side of the wrist. LT injury can be clinically encountered in athletes participating in high-energy/impact sports such as football, hockey, rugby, and basketball.[1] LT injury presents within a spectrum of severity, similar to scapholunate (SL) injuries, and injury can range from isolated membranous tears to frank dislocation. Several different mechanisms of injury have been described, including dorsally applied forces, ulnar positive variance, and perilunate/reverse perilunate injury patterns. Patients present complaining of ulnar-sided wrist pain and decreased grip strength. Successful treatment of LT injury is predicated on the proper index of suspicion, precise diagnosis, the chronicity with which the injury presents, and the assessment of the degree of carpal instability. For the specific treatment of acute LT injuries, options include steroid injection, immobilization, arthroscopic debridement, and open ligament repair. Chronically presenting injuries are managed with ligament reconstruction using tendon grafts, limited intercarpal fusions, and ulnar shortening.

PATHOMECHANICS

The LTIL stabilizes the LT joint.[2] The LTIL, like the SL ligament, is made up of 3 regions, a dorsal, membranous, and volar region. The volar region of the LTIL is the most stout and is considered the major constraint to LT motion. There are several extrinsic ligaments that help to further stabilize the LT relationship; these include the palmar radiolunotriquetral ligament and the dorsal radiocarpal ligament.

It is important to understand the triquetrum's role in carpal mechanics to understand the problems that develop after LT injury. The triquetrum links the distal carpal row to the proximal carpal role through its articulation with the hamate. During radial deviation, the scaphoid is pushed into

Dr M.C. Nicoson has nothing to disclose. Dr S.L. Moran is a consultant for Integra, Conventus, and Axogen.
[a] Hand and Wrist of Louisville, 2400 Eastpoint Parkway, Suite 570, Louisville, KY 40223, USA; [b] Division of Plastic Surgery, Mayo Clinic, 200 1st Street Southwest, Rochester, MN 55901, USA
* Corresponding author.
E-mail address: moran.steven@mayo.edu

Hand Clin 31 (2015) 467–476
http://dx.doi.org/10.1016/j.hcl.2015.04.005
0749-0712/15/$ – see front matter © 2015 Elsevier Inc. All rights reserved.

hand.theclinics.com

flexion by the distal carpal row and pulls the lunate and triquetrum into flexion through an intact scapholunate interosseous ligament (SLIL). During ulnar deviation, the exerted extension force on the triquetrum pulls the rest of the proximal carpal row into extension through and intact LTIL. In radial and ulnar deviation, the motion of the proximal carpal row is the inverse of the distal carpal row; in radial deviation, the distal carpal row moves radially, extends, and supinates, whereas the proximal carpal row flexes and translates ulnarly. During ulnar deviation of the wrist, the distal carpal row moves ulnarly, flexes, and pronates, whereas the proximal carpal row extends and translates radially. The lunate, with its interosseous attachments to the SLIL and LTIL, tends to remain balanced because of the opposing forces between the 2 flanking bones (3). With disruption of either the SLIL or LTIL, the lunate is pulled in the direction of the intact ligament, palmar with an intact SLIL and dorsal with and intact LTIL. Over time this instability leads to attritional changes in the secondary stabilizers of the wrist, resulting in abnormal contact between the carpal bones; this may result in the development of a volar (or palmar) intercalated segment instability (VISI) deformity of the proximal row (43). A static VISI deformity implies disruption of the secondary ligamentous constraints of LT motion in addition to disruption of the LTIL.

A complete LT ligament tear alone is not sufficient to cause the carpus to assume a VISI stance. Sectioning of volar and dorsal LT ligaments results in a slight divergence of the triquetrum and lunate at extremes of wrist flexion and radial deviation, but VISI collapse is not apparent unless considerable compressive forces are applied.[2] Additional tears or attenuation of secondary restraints is necessary to result in a static carpal instability. Both palmar and dorsal carpal ligaments likely play a role as secondary restraints. Anatomic studies have implicated palmar ligament injury in the development of VISI in LT dissociation. Trumble and colleagues[3] created carpal collapse with division of the ulnar arcuate ligament, whereas Viegas and colleagues[4] and Ritt and colleagues[5,6] found the palmar LT ligament to be the thickest and strongest when tested to mechanical failure. The dorsal LT ligament serves mainly as a rotational constraint. LT ligament disruption leads to an increase in the moment arm of the flexor carpi ulnaris tendon that may contribute to additional clinical sequelae seen in patients.[7]

Sectioning of the dorsal radiocarpal and intercarpal ligament produces a static VISI stance following LT ligament injury.[5,6,8] Loss of dorsal ligament integrity allows the lunate to flex more easily

in part by shifting the point of capitate contact palmar to the lunate axis of rotation. Although LT ligament dissociation can result in a VISI deformity, not all VISI deformities are the result of LT ligament injury. Carpal instability of the nondissociative type of the radiocarpal, midcarpal, or combined radiocarpal-midcarpal joints can also lead to VISI deformity.[9]

The language used in the description of LT ligament injuries should be precise; it is important to distinguish between dynamic and static forms of instability. LT ligament injuries with normal findings on conventional radiographs and dynamic instability (visible only under load) are classified as LT attenuations or tears. Fixed carpal collapse (VISI) on conventional radiographs represents static instability and is classified as LT ligament dissociation.

MECHANISM OF INJURY
Dorsally Applied Force

Weber postulated that isolated LT tears may occur when a dorsally applied force is applied to a palmarly flexed wrist.[10] The dorsal force can result in the dorsal LT interosseous fibers to fail, sparing the palmar radiolunotriquetral ligaments (**Fig. 1**). The integrity of this ligament tethers the palmar pole of the lunate, therein leading to an axis of palmarly directed flexion.

Perilunate Injury

The entity and mechanism of isolated LT ligament injury remains a topic of debate and is less well understood than SLIL injury. It is likely that multiple mechanisms play supporting causative roles. For example, perilunate dislocations occur when forces are applied to the thenar area with the wrist in a position of dorsiflexion and ulnar deviation.[11–15] The resulting intercarpal supination leads to a progressive injury pattern from a radial to ulnar direction (**Fig. 2**), following either a bony or purely

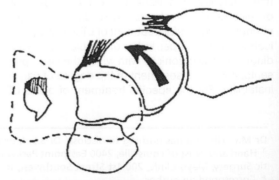

Fig. 1. Dorsal radiocarpal tear. (By permission of the Mayo Foundation for Medical Education and Research. All rights reserved.)

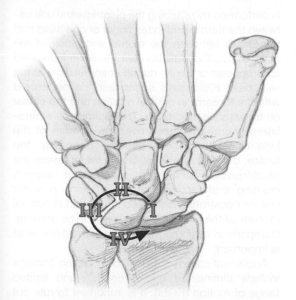

ligamentous corridor about the lunate. Mayfield stage III is the specific stage of injury to the LT support structures, which follows injury to the SL or scaphoid proper from a fracture. These injuries typically lead to a dorsal intercalated segment instability deformity, except in situations in which the SL ligament heals spontaneously or with intervention.[16,17] In such instances, ulnar-sided pathology predominates.

Reverse Perilunate Injury

The presence of an isolated LT tear may represent a reverse pattern of the perilunate injury (**Fig. 3**) originating on the ulnar side of the wrist.[2,17,18] Biomechanical studies have confirmed this mechanism, which likely occurs from falling on the outstretched hand with the wrist positioned in extension, pronation, and radial deviation. The resultant intercarpal pronation overloads the ulnar-volar ligament structures, therein leading to an LT ligament injury, without affecting the SLIL complex.

Other Causes

Patients without an antecedent history of trauma may have degenerative LT lesions or inflammatory arthritis that leads to LT instability.[19,20] Radiographic findings of ulnar abutment can facilitate LT membrane degeneration either by a wear mechanism or by altering intercarpal kinematics.[21–25]

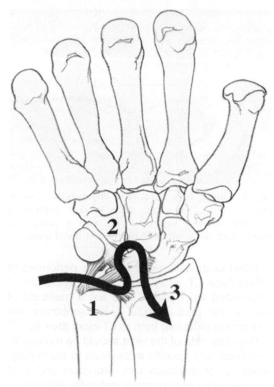

EVALUATION OF LUNOTRIQUETRAL INJURIES

LT ligament injury evaluation is challenging because of the range of clinical presentation. Patients with partial LT tears present with variable pain and grip weakness. Complete LT dissociation presents with static collapse causing a forklike deformity of the wrist (**Fig. 4**) and distal ulna prominence.[17,26] Some patients with radiographic evidence of persistent LT malalignment after perilunate dislocation may have minimal symptoms and a satisfactory outcome.[27,28] LT sprains that are symptomatic present invariably with intermittent ulnar-sided wrist pain that is noticeable with wrist deviation.[2,26] Patients present with weakness, diminished motion, sensations of instability or giving way, and ulnar nerve paresthesias. On physical examination, it is common to see a painful wrist clunk with wrist deviation.[2]

Obtaining a detailed history is crucial and typically reveals the mechanism and the specific injury.[2] History of falling on the dorsiflexed wrist with a hypothenar contact point should increase the suspicion of ulnar-sided instability.[29] Next, a

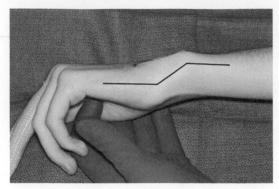

Fig. 4. Dinner fork deformity. Preoperative clinical image of a 25-year-old male worker presenting 6 weeks after a sustained fall with a prominent dinner-fork deformity and prominent distal ulna.

detailed examination of the wrist is performed to differentiate LT injury from other generators of ulnar-sided wrist pain. There are a multitude of lesions that cause medial wrist symptoms that distract the examiner from an LT injury (**Box 1**).[30,31]

The ulnar side of the wrist should be thoroughly examined with specific maneuvers to aid in diagnosis. Ulnar deviation with pronation and axial compression elicits dynamic instability with a painful snap if a nondissociative midcarpal or LT injury is present. Direct palpation of the LT joint always results in point tenderness.[2,17] Provocative tests, including the LT ballottement; compression; and shear test[2,29,32] are useful in accurately localizing the site of pathology and clinically result in LT laxity, crepitus, and pain on examination.

Triquetral compression in the ulnar snuff box applies a radially directed compressive force against the triquetrum. Pain elicited from this maneuver may be of LT origin but may also develop from the triquetrohamate joint or triangular fibrocartilagenous complex (TFCC).[29] Triquetrum ballottement, as described by Reagan and colleagues,[2]

Box 1
Generators of ulnar-sided wrist pain

Ulnar impaction syndrome

Traumatic or degenerative tears of the TFCC

Kienböck disease

Triquetral avulsion fractures

Pisotriquetral arthritis

Extensor carpi ulnaris subluxation or tenosynovitis

Entrapment of the dorsal cutaneous branch of the ulnar nerve

Distal radioulnar joint subluxation or arthrosis

is performed by grasping the pisotriquetral unit between the thumb and index finger of one hand and the lunate between the thumb and index of the other. A positive ballottement results in increased anteroposterior laxity during manipulation along with pain. Kleinman's shear test[32] is performed with the forearm in neutral rotation and the elbow on the examination table. The examiner's contralateral thumb is placed over the dorsum of the lunate. While simultaneously supporting the lunate, the examiner's ipsilateral thumb loads the pisotriquetral joint from the palmar aspect, creating a shear force at the LT joint. A shear test demonstrating pain, crepitance, and abnormal mobility of the LT joint is considered to be positive. Comparison of finding with the contralateral wrist is important.

Additional salient physical examination findings include diminished grip strength[17] and limited range of motion (ROM). It is important to rule out a nondissociative instability pattern secondary to midcarpal laxity at the triquetrohamate joint as symptoms may be similar and there is the possibility of injury at both levels.[16,31,33]

IMAGING STUDIES

Diagnostic studies are beneficial in the evaluation of LT injuries. Standard posteroanterior and lateral views of the wrist in neutral rotation are critical for all patients complaining of ulnar-sided wrist pain. Additional relevant investigations include motion studies, tomography, arthrography, videofluoroscopy, scintigraphy, and MRI.

Radiographs of wrist with LT tears frequently show normal findings (**Fig. 5**). LT dissociation results in a disruption of Gilula arc I and II, with proximal translation of the triquetrum and/or LT overlap.[2,34] In contradistinction to SL injuries, LT gapping rarely occurs. A static VISI deformity implies not only direct injury to the LT ligament but also additional dorsal or palmar ligament attenuation.[2–4,8] Motion studies, including deviation and clenched fist anteroposterior views are often helpful. In LT dissociation, the normal reciprocal motion of the scaphoid, lunate, and distal row is accentuated in deviation with diminished triquetral motion.[29]

Careful review of lateral radiographs is useful to detect VISI deformity and also to reveal relative malalignment between the lunate and triquetrum in the absence of frank carpal collapse.[17] The perimeters of the triquetrum and lunate may be traced out to assist in their relational assessment.[2,17] The normal triquetrolunate angle is 14° (range +31° to −3°), but Reagan and colleagues[2] found this to be a negative angle (mean value

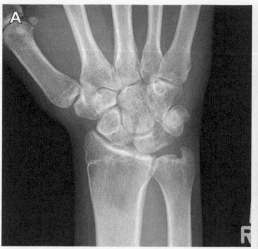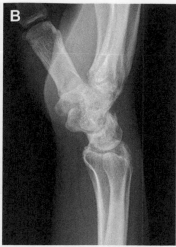

Fig. 5. Radiographs of LT injury. (*A*) Posteroanterior radiograph of same patient described in **Fig. 4** with disruption of Gilula arcs I and II, with proximal migration of the triquetrum relative to the lunate. (*B*) Lateral radiograph showing volar intercalated segment instability with abnormal flexion of the lunate.

−16°) with LT dissociation. If a VISI deformity is present in conjunction with LT dissociation, SL and capitolunate angles are both altered. The SL angle is diminished from its normal 47° to 40°or less.[35–37] The normally colinear lunate and capitate collapse in a zigzag manner, resulting in an angle greater than 10°.

Arthrography historically was helpful to diagnose LT tears and demonstrate dye leakage at the LT interspace; however, arthrograms can be read as abnormal in the ulnar-positive wrist, as age-related LT membrane perforations are common,[19,38] with 13% of normal individuals showing communication of radiocarpal and midcarpal joints.[39–41] In a cadaver study, Viegas and colleagues[42] were able to demonstrate that 36% of wrist dissections had evidence of LT tears. Cantor and colleagues[43] also found that 59% of patients with unilateral wrist symptoms and an LT tear on arthrography demonstrated similar arthrographic findings in the asymptomatic wrist. This finding highlights the importance of careful interpretation of arthrography findings and correlating the findings with a detailed clinical examination.

Historically, videoarthrography with motion sequences in flexion-extension and radial-ulnar deviation could confirm the presence of an LT injury by demonstration of abnormal dye column pooling and abnormal proximal row kinematics.[44,45] Videofluoroscopy is useful in demonstrating the site of a clunk that occurs with deviation. In LT sprains, this occurs with a sudden catch-up extension of the triquetrum as the wrist moves into maximal ulnar deviation.

Other imaging studies may be useful at times. Technetium Tc 99m methylene diphosphonate

bone scans can help identify the site of acute injury but are less specific than arthrography.[34] They may prove helpful in cases in which standard films and motion studies show negative findings. MRI technology (**Fig. 6**) is not yet reliable for LT ligament imaging.[46] Negative results on magnetic resonance (MR) studies for LT injury does not rule out the presence of pathology, as not all MR studies adequately detect LT lesions.[24] MR arthrography has replaced historic arthrograms in many centers; however, its specificity and sensitivity for LT injury has yet to be clearly defined.

Most surgeons still find wrist arthroscopy to serve as the gold standard for the diagnosis of LT injury (**Fig. 7**). Wrist arthroscopy serves a dual role for both diagnosis and therapeutic intervention.[24,47,48] Arthroscopic inspection provides an

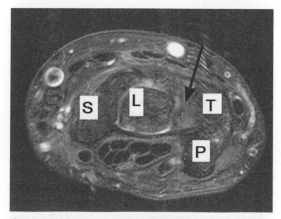

Fig. 6. MRI is not always reliable for LT injury. However, LT tears can be seen, typically in the presence of large area of edema surrounding the joint (*arrow*). L, lunate; P, pisiform; S, scaphoid; T, triquetrum.

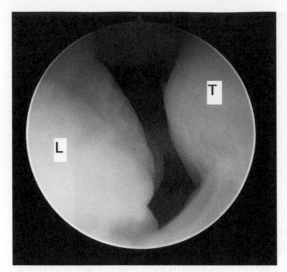

Fig. 7. Wrist arthroscopy for LT pathology. Intraoperative arthroscopic image revealing a Geissler grade IV tear of the LT ligament from the 4,5 viewing portal. L, lunate; T, triquetrum.

avenue for direct evaluation of the LT ligament and assessment for instability and disruption. It has been the authors' experience that arthroscopy provides the most accurate means of diagnosis of LT pathology and should be considered for cases of high clinical suspicion but negative MRI findings.

CLASSIFICATION

Viegas and colleagues[4] described the following classification of LT ligament injury:

Grade 1: Partial or incomplete LT tear without VISI deformity
Grade 2: Complete LT ligament tear with lesion of the palmar ligaments and dynamic VISI deformity
Grade 3: Complete LT ligament tear with lesion of the palmar and dorsal ligaments and static VISI deformity

TREATMENT

Choosing the optimal treatment of LT injury requires consideration of multiple factors, including the amount of instability (static vs dynamic), the elapsed time between injury and treatment, and the presence of associated injury or degenerative changes. Symptoms of pain in LT attenuations or tears may be due to dynamic instability and/or local synovitis.[16]

Initial management of partial isolated LT injuries without dissociation should be nonoperative, with cast or splint immobilization above the elbow.[2,26,29,34,36] Careful splint molding with a

pad underneath the pisiform maintains optimal alignment as ligamentous healing progresses. Nonsteroidal anti-inflammatory medications may be prescribed. Corticosteroid injections into the midcarpal joint can also be helpful in decreasing synovitis. Typically, a 6-week period of immobilization alone is adequate to allow intrinsic healing of the LT ligament.

For acute injuries presenting with instability and tears unresponsive to conservative management, operative intervention is warranted. The goal of operative intervention is the realignment of the lunocapitate axis and reestablishment of the rotational integrity of the proximal carpal row.[10,49] Arthroscopic intervention and treatment of LT tears has been gaining interest and in some cases is used a first-line modality in certain patient cohorts, such as high-level athletes.

An arthroscopic evaluation of the radiocarpal and midcarpal joints is performed and LT instability confirmed. Any associated injury is noted for arthroscopic or open repair. The LT ligament is best visualized from the 4-5, 6R, and midcarpal portals. It is essential that dorsal, volar, and membranous portions of the LT ligament are visualized and palpated with a probe to ascertain the integrity of the ligament. Midcarpal arthroscopy is the key to assessing the stability of the LT joint.[50] From the midcarpal perspective, the normal LT joint is smooth without a step-off or diastasis.[51] Placement of a probe into the LT allows one to assess for any dynamic instability. The degree of ligament injury is classified by the arthroscopic classification of tears of the intracarpal ligaments as described by Geissler and colleagues[52] (**Table 1**). In addition to inspection of the LT joint, arthroscopy aids in the identification of concomitant injuries such as TFCC tears or arthritic changes to the articular surfaces of the hamate, triquetrum, capitates, and lunate.

For acute lesions of the LT ligament, an arthroscopic motorized shaver is used to carefully debride the frayed ligamentous edges to a stable margin and promote healing. In cases in which there is no instability, arthroscopic debridement alone can be successful.[53] Weiss and colleagues[53] noted that 100% of patients with a partial LT tear and 78% with a complete tear had symptom resolution. Possibility of performing an arthroscopic reduction of the LT joint is then assessed using the midcarpal portal. This procedure is facilitated by using Kirschner (K) wire joysticks into the lunate and triquetrum or the arthroscopic probe. For Geissler grade II and III lesions, K-wire fixation (two or three 0.045 in) is then performed from the triquetrum into the lunate, and the pins are buried subcutaneously. The wrist

Table 1 Arthroscopic classification of the tears of the intracarpal ligaments	
Grade	Description
I	Attenuation or hemorrhage of the interosseous ligament as seen from the radiocarpal space. No incongruency of carpal alignment in the midcarpal space
II	Attenuation or hemorrhage of interosseous ligament as seen from the radiocarpal space. Incongruency or step-off of carpal space. There may be slight gap (less than width of probe) between carpal bones
III	Incongruency or step-off of carpal alignment as seen from both radiocarpal and midcarpal space. Probe may be passed through gap between carpal bones
IV	Incongruency or step-off of carpal alignment as seen from both radiocarpal and midcarpal space. There is gross instability with manipulation. A 2.7-mm arthroscope may be passed through the gap between carpal bones

From Geissler WB, Freeland AE, Savoie FH, et al. Intracarpal soft-tissue lesions associated with an intra-articular fracture of the distal end of the radius. J Bone Joint Surg Am 1996;78(3):357–65.

is subsequently immobilized for 8 weeks, and then the pins are removed.

For Geissler grade IV acute lesions of the LT ligament, direct repair is necessary. Following arthroscopy, a curvilinear incision is made distal to the ulnocarpal articulation. The dorsal branch of the ulnar nerve is identified and protected. The extensor retinaculum is divided over the extensor pollicis longus, developing retinacular flaps by division of the septae over separating the second through the fifth extensor compartments. A posterior interosseous neurectomy is performed to partially denervate the dorsal wrist capsule. The dorsal radiotriquetral and scaphotriquetral (dorsal radiocarpal and intercarpal) ligaments are identified, and a capsulotomy is made as described by Berger and Bishop.[54] The midcarpal and radiocarpal joint surfaces are exposed and examined for arthritic changes. The SL and LT ligaments are thoroughly examined (**Fig. 8**).

For open primary LT repair there are 2 options. The ligament may be reconstructed through drill holes or with the aid of suture anchors. The bone hole technique proceeds as follows: The ligament remnant is freshened, and the site of avulsion from

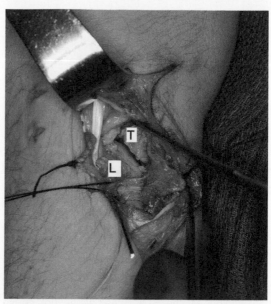

Fig. 8. Operative approach to the LT joint. Surgical exposure of the LT joint reveals injury to the entire dorsal portion of the LTIL, with resultant diastasis. L, lunate; T, triquetrum.

the triquetrum is prepared by abrading the bone surface. About 3 to 4 parallel holes are placed in this side exiting dorsally using a 0.028-in K-wire. About 2 to 3 sets of nonabsorbable sutures (3-0) are passed through the drill holes, into the LT ligament and back through the drill holes (**Figs. 9** and **10**). A

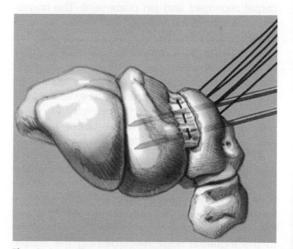

Fig. 9. Lunotriquetral ligament repair. Diagram of ligament repair using bone hole technique. Parallel holes are placed across the triquetrum to the triquetral lunate joint. The radial surface of the triquetrum is freshened to encourage bone healing. Kirschner wires are placed from ulnar to radial across the LT joint, and the sutures are tied. (By permission of the Mayo Foundation for Medical Education and Research. All rights reserved.)

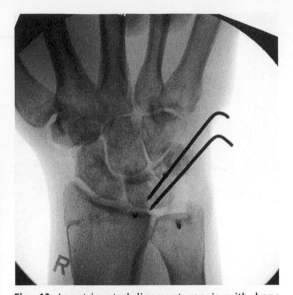

Fig. 10. Lunotriquetral ligament repair with bone anchor. Postreduction radiograph showing a reduced LT interval, stabilized with 2 Kirschner wires and a single bone anchor in the triquetrum. The suture is passed through the remaining LTIL and tied down to the triquetrum. Note that there is an additional visualized anchor for TFCC repair.

Keith needle with 4-0 Prolene suture assists with the placement of the suture through the drill holes. About 2 to 3 K-wires, 0.045 in, are passed percutaneously through the triquetrum and lunate in a reduced position. Radiographs then confirm proper carpal alignment and pin placement. The nonabsorbable sutures are then tied and the dorsal radiotriquetral ligament portion of the capsular flap sutured to the repair, providing additional augmentation. The remaining capsular flap is repaired and the extensor retinaculum reapproximated with absorbable sutures, transposing the extensor pollicis longus tendon dorsal to the retinaculum.

If suture anchors are to be used, they are routinely placed over the dorsal surface of the triquetrum. K-wires are passed transcutaneously through the triquetrum and into a reduced lunate. Once the joint is reduced, the sutures are passed through the remaining LT ligament and tied down to the triquetrum. The sutures are left long and then used to secure the capsular flap back down to the triquetral ridge reestablishing the attachment for the dorsal intercarpal ligament. The K-wires are removed at 8 weeks. Volar repair may be required if the triquetrum is significantly supinated in relation to the lunate or if the volar ligament has sustained a significant tear as in a perilunate dislocation.

Repair of the LT ligament has been described by several investigators.[2,55,56] Reagan and

colleagues[2] demonstrated good results, as did Shin and colleagues.[57,58] The LTIL is reattached to the site of its avulsion, generally to the triquetrum. If the palmar ligament is also disrupted, a combined dorsal and palmar approach may be necessary. Augmentation of the repair by dorsal capsulodesis and dorsal ligament repair may also be of some value. Protracted immobilization is necessary as for SL ligament repairs. Patients with strenuous pursuits, chronic instability, or poor-quality LT ligament may be best managed by ligament reconstruction.

COMPLICATIONS

Complications can be minimized by careful attention to detail, including protection of the dorsal sensory branch of the ulnar nerve (DSBUN), correction of the VISI deformity before ligament repair or reconstruction, and care in creation of bone tunnels. The only complication seen postoperatively in Shin and colleagues'[57] review of reconstruction was DSBUN neuritis, and of repairs, there was a 14.8% failure rate (secondary to recurrent injury) and DSBUN neuritis.

REHABILITATION

Active and passive ROM exercises of the fingers, elbow, and shoulder, as well as antiedema measures, may be begun immediately. The postoperative dressing and sutures are removed between 10 and 14 days postoperatively, and a long arm cast in neutral forearm rotation placed for 6 to 8 weeks.

The pins are removed at 8 to 10 weeks after ligament repair, and the wrist is supported with a splint during the rehabilitation period. Strengthening exercises are begun once ROM has returned. The wrist can be supported with a splint during activities for an additional 3 to 6 months. Longer periods of immobilization have been recommended and may be beneficial in more severe injuries, although there are no good long-term studies examining postoperative immobilization patterns in LT injuries; however, postoperative stiffness has been correlated with successful outcomes.[47,57,59,60]

Pins are removed between 8 and 12 weeks after ligament reconstruction, and gentle ROM of the wrist is initiated with periodic splinting for an additional 8 weeks. Strengthening and increasing ROM exercises continue during this period.

SUMMARY

Treatment of acutely presenting LT injuries remains a topic of debate, and many avenues of intervention are available. LT tears are uncommon, and the available evidence is limited to retrospective case reviews. Based on experience and the available literature, for acute presenting cases without instability, the authors recommend 6 weeks of immobilization. For acute cases with instability, they recommend wrist arthroscopy with or without pinning, with direct repair of the LT ligament for full-thickness lesions. Although surgical repair can be technically challenging, it preserves LT motion and provides the optimal chance for restoration of normal carpal interactions.

REFERENCES

1. Linscheid RL, Dobyns JH. Athletic injuries of the wrist. Clin Orthop Relat Res 1985;(198):141–51.
2. Reagan DS, Linscheid RL, Dobyns JH. Lunotriquetral Sprains. J Hand Surg 1984;9A(4):502–14.
3. Trumble TE, Bour CJ, Smith RJ, et al. Kinematics of the ulnar carpus related to the volar intercalated segment instability pattern. J Hand Surg 1990; 15A(3):384–92.
4. Viegas SF, Patterson RM, Peterson PD, et al. Ulnar sided perilunate instability: an anatomic and biomechanic study. J Hand Surg 1990;15A(2):268–78.
5. Ritt MJ, Bishop AT, Berger RA, et al. Lunotriquetral ligament properties: a comparison of three anatomic subregions. J Hand Surg 1998;23A:425–31.
6. Ritt MJ, Linscheid RL, Cooney WP 3rd, et al. The lunotriquetral joint: kinematic effects of sequential ligament sectioning, ligament repair and arthrodesis. J Hand Surg 1998;23A:432–45.
7. Tang JB, Xie RG, Yu XW, et al. Wrist kinematics after luno-triquetral dissociation: the change in the moment arms of the flexor carpi ulnaris tendon. J Orthop Res 2002;20(6):1327–32.
8. Horii E, Garcia-Elias M, An KN, et al. A kinematic study of luno-triquetral dissociations. J Hand Surg 1991;16A(2):355–62.
9. Dobyns JH, Cooney WP 3rd. Classification of carpal instability. In: Cooney WP 3rd, Linscheid RL, Dobyns JH, editors. The wrist: diagnosis and operative treatment. St Louis (MO): Mosby; 1997. p. 490–500.
10. Weber ERA. Wrist mechanics and its association with ligamentous instability. In: Lichtman DM, editor. The wrist and its disorders. Philadelphia: WB Saunders; 1988. p. 41–52.
11. Johnson RP. The acutely injured wrist and its residuals. Clin Orthop Relat Res 1980;(149):33–44.
12. Mayfield JK. Patterns of injury to carpal ligaments - a spectrum. Clin Orthop Relat Res 1984;(187):36–42.
13. Mayfield JK, Johnson RP, Kilcoyne RF. The ligaments of the wrist and their functional significance. Anat Rec 1976;186:417–28.
14. Mayfield JK, Johnson RP, Kilcoyne RK. Pathomechanics and progressive perilunar instability. J Hand Surg 1980;5A:226–41.
15. McAuliffe JA, Dell PC, Jaffe R. Complications of intercarpal arthrodesis. J Hand Surg 1993;18A(6): 1121–8.
16. Lichtman DM, Noble WH, Alexander CE. Dynamic triquetrolunate instability: case report. J Hand Surg 1984;9A:185–7.
17. Linscheid RL, Dobyns JH. The unified concept of carpal injuries. Ann Chir Main 1984;3:35–42.
18. Murray PM, Palmer CG, Shin AY. The mechanism of ulnar-sided perilunate instability of the wrist: a cadaveric study and 6 clinical cases. J Hand Surg Am 2012;37(4):721–8.
19. Mikic ZD. Arthrography of the wrist joint. An experimental study. J Bone Joint Surg Am 1984;66:371–4.
20. Taleisnik J, Malerich M, Prietto M. Palmar carpal instability secondary to dislocation of scaphoid and lunate: report of case and review of the literature. J Hand Surg 1982;7A(6):606–12.
21. Palmer AK, Glisson RR, Werner W. Relationship between ulnar variance and triangular fibrocartilage complex thickness. J Hand Surg 1984;9A:681–3.
22. Palmer AK, Werner RW. Biomechanics of the distal radioulnar joint. Clin Orthop Relat Res 1984;(187): 26–35.
23. Pin PG, Young VL, Gilula LA, et al. Management of chronic lunotriquetral ligament tears. J Hand Surg 1989;14A(1):77–83.
24. Weiss LE, Taras JS, Sweet S, et al. Lunotriquetral injuries in the athlete. Hand Clin 2000;16(3):433–8.
25. Werner FW, Glisson RR, Murphy DJ, et al. Force transmission through the distal radioulnar carpal joint: the effect of ulnar lengthening and shortening. Handchirurgie, Mikrochirurgie. Z Plast Chir 1986; 15(5):304–8.
26. Culver JE. Instabilities of the wrist. Clin Sports Med 1986;5(4):725–40.
27. Minami A, Ogino T, Ohshio I, et al. Correlation between clinical results and carpal instabilities in patients after reduction of lunate and perilunate dislocations. J Hand Surg 1986;11B:213–20.
28. Nelson DL, Manske PR, Pruitt DL, et al. Lunotriquetral arthrodesis. J Hand Surg 1993;18A(6): 1113–20.
29. Beckenbaugh RD. Accurate evaluation and management of the painful wrist following injury. Orthop Clin North Am 1984;15(2):289–306.
30. Bishop AT. The dilemma of ulnar sided wrist pain. Prob Plast Reconstr Surg 1992;2:199–213.
31. Lichtman DM, Schneider JR, Swafford AR, et al. Ulnar midcarpal instability - clinical and laboratory analysis. J Hand Surg 1981;6A(5):515–23.
32. Kleinman WB. Diagnostic exams for ligamentous injuries. Am Soc Surg Hand, Correspondence Club Newsletter 1985;51.

33. Trumble T, Bour CJ, Smith RJ, et al. Intercarpal arthrodesis for static and dynamic volar intercalated segment instability. J Hand Surg 1988;13A:384–90.

34. Gilula LA, Weeks PM. Post-traumatic ligamentous instabilities of the wrist. Radiology 1978;129(3):641–51.

35. Linscheid RL, Dobyns JH, Beabout JW, et al. Traumatic instability of the wrist. Diagnosis, classification and pathomechanics. J Bone Joint Surg Am 1972;54:1612–32.

36. Sebald JR, Dobyns JH, Linscheid RL. The natural history of collapse deformity of the wirst. Clin Orthop 1974;104:140–8.

37. Sennwald GR, Fischer M, Mondi P. Lunotriquetral arthrodesis. A controversial procedure. J Hand Surg 1995;20B(6):755–60.

38. Trentham DE, Hamm RE, Madi AT. Wrist arthrography: review and comparison of normals, rheumatoid arthritis and gout patients. Semin Arthritis Rheum 1975;5:105–20.

39. Kessler I, Silberman Z. An experimental study of the radiocarpal joint by arthrography. Surg Gynecol Obstet 1961;112:33.

40. Kirschenbaum D, Coyle MP, Leddy JP. Chronic lunotriquetral instability: diagnosis and treatment. J Hand Surg 1993;18A(6):1107–12.

41. Kricun ME. Wrist arthrography. Clin Orthop Relat Res 1984;(187):64–71.

42. Viegas SF, Patterson RM, Hokanson JA, et al. Wrist anatomy: incidence, distribution, and correlation of anatomic variations, tears and arthrosis. J Hand Surg 1993;18A:463–75.

43. Cantor RM, Stern PJ, Wyrick JD, et al. The relevance of ligament tears or perforations in the diagnosis of wrist pain: an arthrographic study. J Hand Surg 1994;19A(6):945–53.

44. Levinsohn EM, Palmer AK. Arthrography of the traumatized wrist. Correlation with radiography and the carpal instability series. Radiology 1983;146(3):647–51.

45. Schwartz AM, Ruby LK. Wrist arthrography revisited. Orthopedics 1982;5:883–8.

46. Yu JS. MRI techniques and practical applications: MRI of the wrist. Orthopedics 1994;17:1041–8.

47. Osterman AL, Seidman GD. The role of arthroscopy in the treatment of lunotriquetral ligament injuries. Hand Clin 1995;11(1):41–50.

48. Whipple TL. Precautions for arthroscopy of the wrist. Arthroscopy 1990;6(1):3–4.

49. Taleisnik J. Pain on the ulnar side of the wrist. Hand Clin 1987;3(1):51–68.

50. Hofmeister EP, Dao KD, Glowacki KA, et al. The role of midcarpal arthroscopy in the diagnosis of disorders of the wrist. J Hand Surg 2001;26A(3):407–14.

51. Hanker GJ. Diagnostic and operative arthroscopy of the wrist. Clin Orthop Relat Res 1991;(263):165–74.

52. Geissler WB, Freeland AE, Savoie FH, et al. Intracarpal soft-tissue lesions associated with an intra-articular fracture of the distal end of the radius. J Bone Joint Surg Am 1996;78(3):357–65.

53. Weiss APC, Sachar K, Glowacki KA, et al. Arthroscopic debridement alone for intercarpal ligament tears. J Hand Surg Am 1997;22:344–9.

54. Berger RA, Bishop AT. A fiber-splitting capsulotomy technique for dorsal exposure of the wrist. Tech Hand Up Extrem Surg 1997;1(1):2–10.

55. Favero KJ, Bishop AT, Linscheid RL. Lunotriquetral ligament disruption: a comparative study of treatment methods (abstract SS-80). Presented at the 46th Annual Meeting of the American Society for Surgery of the Hand. Orlando, FLA October 2-5, 1991.

56. Palmer AK, Dobyns JH, Linscheid RL. Management of post-traumatic instability of the wrist secondary to ligament rupture. J Hand Surg 1978;3A:507–32.

57. Shin AY, Weinstein LP, Berger RA, et al. Treatment of isolated injuries of the lunotriquetral ligament. A comparison of arthrodesis, ligament reconstruction and ligament repair. J Bone Joint Surg Br 2001;83(7):1023–8.

58. Simmons BP, McKenzie WD. Symptomatic carpal coalition. J Hand Surg 1985;10A:190–3.

59. Shin AY, Battaglia MJ, Bishop AT. Lunotriquetral instability: diagnosis and treatment. J Am Acad Orthop Surg 2000;8(3):170–9.

60. Shin AY, Bishop AT. Treatment options for lunotriquetral dissociation. Tech Hand Upper Extremity Surg 1998;2(1):2–17.

Diagnosis and Treatment of Chronic Lunotriquetral Ligament Injuries

Eric R. Wagner, MD, Bassem T. Elhassan, MD,
Marco Rizzo, MD*

KEYWORDS

- Wrist • Ligament • Lunotriquetral • Reconstruction • Arthrodesis • Ulnar shortening

KEY POINTS

- Chronic lunotriquetral (LT) injuries are rare and often difficult to diagnose.
- Plain radiographs are often normal and ancillary studies, such as MRI, are used when working up these cases.
- Direct visualization of the LT interval remains the gold standard for evaluating ligament injuries.
- Surgical treatment options for chronic lunotriquetral injuries include reconstruction and arthrodesis.
- Ulnar-shortening osteotomy may be helpful in cases of concomitant ulnocarpal impingement.

INTRODUCTION

The C-shaped lunotriquetral (LT) interosseous ligament works with the scapholunate (SL) interosseous ligament to stabilize the proximal carpal row. The proximal carpal row stability is associated with an equilibrium of forces on the lunate, between the extension moment of the triquetrum (transmitted through the LT ligament) and the flexion moment of the scaphoid (transmitted through the SL ligament). Unlike the SL ligament, where the dorsal aspect is the most critical, the thick volar LT ligament is associated with the ulnocapitate ligament to act as the major stabilizing force, transmitting the extension moment of the triquetrum when it engages the triquetrum.[1] The dorsal LT ligament is not as strong, acting to stabilize rotational forces through the proximal row. Furthermore, there are other secondary restraints to the LT complex stability, such as the radiotriquetral, radioscapholunate, and radiolunate ligaments.

LT ligament injuries are not as well understood as their counterpart SL ligament. LT ligament injuries can occur in isolation, but often are associated with other wrist trauma, including distal radius fractures or perilunate dislocations. One proposed mechanism that induces an LT injury involves a fall on a pronated wrist with the wrist in either radial deviation or volar flexion.[2] Furthermore, positive ulnar variance leading to ulnocarpal impingement can alter wrist intercarpal mechanics and lead to LT ligament degeneration.[3,4]

LUNOTRIQUETRAL DISSOCIATIVE INSTABILITY

The key component of the LT ligament complex is the volar aspect of the ligament. This was demonstrated by Ritt and colleagues,[1] where serial sectioning of the dorsal LT ligament had little effect on carpal kinematics, and sectioning the proximal and volar LT ligament led to flexion of the lunate and subsequent volar intercalated instability (VISI). Complete disruption of the LT ligament is associated with acute trauma or chronic wrist degenerative processes. If left untreated, these

The authors have nothing to disclose.
Department of Orthopedic Surgery, Mayo Clinic, 200 First Street Southwest, Rochester, MN 55905, USA
* Corresponding author.
E-mail address: Rizzo.marco@mayo.edu

Hand Clin 31 (2015) 477–486
http://dx.doi.org/10.1016/j.hcl.2015.04.006

hand.theclinics.com

injuries have the potential to develop dynamic or static carpal instability. Dynamic instability occurs when the LT ligament is partially or completely torn or attenuated, but falls shorts of complete LT dissociation. Complete (dorsal and volar) ligament dissociation may lead to static instability that is able to be diagnosed on plain radiographs. Once the secondary restraints to the LT complex become attenuated, the balance of forces between the scaphoid and triquetrum on the lunate is disrupted, leading to volar flexion of the lunate in conjunction with the scaphoid, also known as VISI (**Fig. 1**). Unlike dorsal intercalated segment instability from complete SL dissociation, the natural history of this pathology and its association with degenerative changes is not well understood.

EXAMINATION AND IMAGING

Chronic ulnar-sided wrist pain has a broad differential diagnosis.[2] The etiologies of chronic ulnar-sided wrist pain tend to involve one of six different categories:

1. Bony injuries: malunions/nonunions of the ulnar carpal bones (hamate, pisiform, triquetrum), base of the fifth metacarpal, ulnar styloid process, and distal ulna.

2. Degenerative joint disease: pisotriquetral, triquetrohamate, fifth carpometacarpal, or distal radioulnar. Degenerative joint disease can be accelerated by ulnar impaction syndrome.

3. Ligamentous (in addition to LT): intrinsic ligaments (capitohamate), extrinsic ligaments (triquetrocapitate or triquetrohamate), triangular fibrocartilage complex.

4. Tendinous: chronic tendinopathy of the extensor carpi ulnaris (ECU) or flexor carpi ulnaris.

5. Neurologic: ulnar nerve entrapment in Guyon canal, neuritis of the dorsal sensory branch of the ulnar nerve.

6. Other: tumors (aneurysmal bone cysts, osteoid osteomas), vascular (ulnar artery thrombosis).

Evaluation of patients with ulnar-sided wrist pain should include a complete upper extremity examination and plain radiographs. In addition, it is not uncommon to obtain advanced diagnostic modalities, such as stress radiographs, computed tomography, ultrasound, bone scan, or MRI. It is helpful to compare with the contralateral unaffected side. Because it may be difficult to discern LT pathology from other conditions that result in ulnar-sided wrist pain, corticosteroid injections in the LT articulations can also be helpful in confirming the diagnosis.

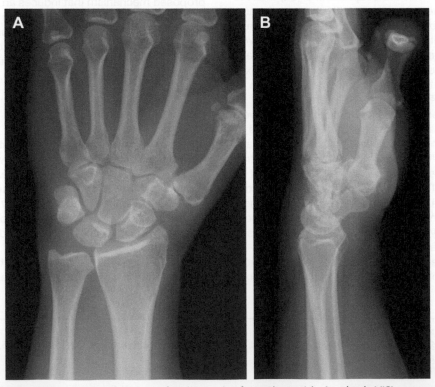

Fig. 1. (*A*) Posteroanterior (PA) and (*B*) lateral radiograph of a patient with the classic VISI.

Pain with palpation on the dorsum of the wrist over the LT interval is highly suggestive of an LT injury.[5] Additional physical examination findings may include a palpable clunk with ulnar deviation and pronation and increased anteroposterior laxity (ballottement test). Another test that elicits pain, crepitance, and abnormal mobility of the LT joint is known as the shear test.[6] Pain with compression of the LT interval from the ulnar aspect of the triquetrum is also suggestive of an LT injury.

Plain radiographs involving the anteroposterior and lateral portions of the wrist should be the first diagnostic modality in a patient with chronic ulnar-sided wrist pain. Static instability and LT dissociation suggest the diagnosis, but unfortunately, the injury may be more subtle. An LT gap becomes apparent, the triquetrum translated proximally, and Gilula I and II arcs are disrupted. Once the extrinsic ligaments become attenuated, a VISI deformity becomes apparent with volar flexion of the lunate. Furthermore, the clenched fist and radial/ulnar deviation views can demonstrate decreased triquetral motion and increased lunate and scaphoid motion.[7]

Another diagnostic maneuver can involve injection of corticosteroid into the LT articulation or the midcarpal space. Other modalities include arthrography to examine for dye leakage into the LT joint or technetium-99m diphosphate bone scan.[7,8] MRI may show abnormalities, but remains relatively nonspecific. Arthroscopy and direct evaluation remain the gold standard for diagnosis.

NONOPERATIVE TREATMENT OF CHRONIC LUNOTRIQUETRAL INJURIES

A patient diagnosed with a subacute or chronic LT tear should be trialed with nonoperative management consisting of immobilization in a splint or cast and anti-inflammatory medications. Unlike acute injuries (where the duration of immobilization is usually 8–12 weeks), the optimal duration for chronic injuries is not known and should be determined by its effectiveness at relieving the patient's symptoms. Of note, in an original study comparing treatment modalities for LT injuries, Reagan and colleagues[5] found chronic LT injuries only responded to immobilization in 25% of patients. However, more recent improvements in conservative treatment strategies have the potential to improve on these findings. Combining immobilization with midcarpal injections likely has the best odds of prolonged improvement of symptoms. Furthermore, Leon-Lopez and colleagues[9] demonstrated that physical therapy targeting ECU strengthening and proprioception has the potential to stabilize the LT joint.

SURGICAL TREATMENT OF CHRONIC LUNOTRIQUETRAL INJURIES

After failure of at least a 3-month trial of nonoperative management, surgical reconstruction or stabilization of the LT articulation can be considered. In static injuries with LT dissociation, surgical success depends on restoring the lunate's "equilibrium" between the scaphoid and triquetrum, stabilizing the proximal carpal row. Surgical options include ligament repair or reconstruction, and LT arthrodesis (**Fig. 2**).[10] Other less commonly used treatments include proximal row carpectomy, denervation, or partial or total wrist arthrodesis in the cases of adjacent joint arthritis. Ulnar shortening osteotomy may be considered in patients with chronic LT instability and concomitant ulnocarpal impingement.[10] Selective neurectomies denervating the dorsal (posterior interosseous) and volar (anterior interosseous) ligaments are also options to treat a patient's pain.[11–13]

The outcome of surgical treatment of chronic LT pathology is not as well elucidated as with the counterpart SL complex. Arthroscopic debridement alone has shown variable outcomes in the treatment of subacute and chronic LT instability.[14,15] Primary repair of the LT ligament has been demonstrated to be successful, especially when the volar ligament remains intact.[4,5,16] In one of the original studies by Reagan and colleagues,[5] six of seven patients underwent LT repairs successfully and led to sustained symptomatic relief. The use of dorsal capsulodesis alone[17–19] or in combination with direct repairs[16] has shown promising results in the chronic setting of dynamic LT instability. Omokawa and colleagues[18] examined 11 patients diagnosed with chronic dynamic LT instability treated with dorsal capsulodesis. At 31 months of follow-up, the patients had significant improvement in their Mayo wrist and pain scores, with maintenance of their range of motion.

In patients with complete tears (volar and dorsal) of the LT ligament, LT reconstruction is a viable option.[2,5,10,16,20] Shahane and colleagues[20] examined 46 patients with chronic posttraumatic LT instability who underwent LT tenodesis with the ECU tendon. At a mean follow-up of 19 months, 19 patients had excellent and 10 had good results, but six patients had poor results and reported they would not undergo the procedure again if given the opportunity. Of note, patients with other wrist pathologies were more likely to have poor results with this technique. Another option for patients with complete tears is LT arthrodesis, with variable results.[5,10,19,21,22] In some of the original studies examining the treatment of chronic LT instability, Kirschenbaum and colleagues[22] and Nelson and

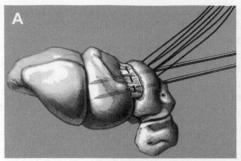
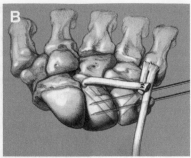
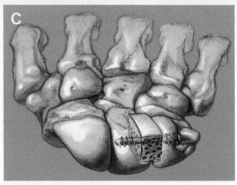

Fig. 2. Schematic drawing of (*A*) primary LT ligament repair, (*B*) LT ligament reconstruction, and (*C*) LT arthrodesis. (By permission of the Mayo Foundation for Medical Education and Research. All rights reserved.)

colleagues[21] demonstrated good pain relief and low rates of short-term complications in 22 and 14 patients, respectively. However, other studies have found high rates of LT nonunion, ulnocarpal impingement, and reoperation, with unpredictable pain relief and overall patient satisfaction in patients undergoing LT arthrodesis.[5,10,19,21]

In a study comparing direct LT repair (N = 27), LT reconstruction with a distally based ECU tenodesis (N = 8), and LT arthrodesis (N = 22), Shin and colleagues[10] examined 57 patients with isolated LT injuries, with most presenting in the chronic setting. The predicted probability of experiencing a 5-year complication was 31% for the reconstructions, compared with 86% for the repairs and 99% for the arthrodeses. Furthermore, the probably of requiring a reoperation was 31% for the reconstruction cohort, compared with 77% for the repairs and 79% for those undergoing arthrodeses. The most common complications in the arthrodesis group included nonunions (41%) and ulnocarpal impaction (23%). There were higher rates of pain relief and satisfaction for those who underwent repair or reconstruction compared with arthrodesis. Furthermore, high-demand patients, such as laborers or athletes, were more likely to experience ligament rerupture after repair.

Other surgical options for patients with LT tears include ulnar-shortening osteotomies, selective denervation, and wrist partial or total fusions.

One option for isolated LT tears in patients with positive ulnar variance and ulnocarpal impingement is an ulnar-shortening osteotomy. The theory behind this procedure is to reduce the abnormal wrist biomechanics produced by ulnar-positive variance, while also tensioning the extrinsic ulnar wrist ligaments to stabilize the LT articulation. In a cadaveric biomechanical study by Gupta and colleagues,[23] the authors demonstrated that ulnar-shortening osteotomies reduced LT strain by tensioning the ulnolunate and ulnotriquetral ligaments. In a clinical study of 53 patients with isolated posttraumatic LT injuries treated with an ulnar-shortening osteotomy, Mirza and colleagues[24] found excellent to good outcomes in 83% of patients, with good pain relief and improvements in grip strengths. A stand-alone or adjunctive surgical option involves selective wrist denervation, including posterior interosseous neurectomy (PIN) and anterior interosseous neurectomy (AIN). Although they have not been evaluated specifically in chronic LT injuries, they have shown promising rates of pain relief in wrist instability and degenerative pathologies.[11–13] Finally, in patients who have degenerative changes in their radiocarpal or midcarpal articulations that are associated with or as result of the LT dissociation, more radical salvage procedures should be considered. If the degenerative changes spare the proximal capitate and lunate fossa, a proximal row carpectomy is an option, whereas four-corner fusion could be considered if the radiolunate articulation is spared. Total wrist fusion should be reserved for patients with pancarpal joint degeneration.

TECHNIQUE: DIAGNOSTIC ARTHROSCOPY, NEURECTOMY, AND LUNOTRIQUETRAL REPAIR (IF POSSIBLE)

If there is any question of the diagnosis or extent of the LT tear, a diagnostic arthroscopy can be performed. A complete evaluation of the LT complex, including the surrounding articular surfaces, ligament integrity, and other associated pathology, can be performed arthroscopically. The surgery is typically performed using a 2.7-mm 30° arthroscope inserted through the radiocarpal (3–4, 4–5, and 6U) and midcarpal (radial and ulnar) portals. Geissler and coworkers[25] classified tears of the LT (similar to the SL) ligament based on arthroscopy from the midcarpal portal as follows:

- Grade I: slight attenuation of the ligament but no visible gap
- Grade II: attenuation of the ligament and a gap between the lunate and triquetrum, but too small to insert a 2-mm probe
- Grade III: disruption of the ligament and a gap large enough to insert a 2-mm probe
- Grade IV: complete disruption of the ligament with a gap large enough to pass through the arthroscope.

Based on the findings of the diagnostic arthroscopy, the surgeon would have one of the following options:

- Partial rupture with intact ligament fibers and pristine articular surfaces: LT repair
- Complete rupture with minimal residual tissue but preserved articular surfaces: LT reconstruction or arthrodesis
- In cases of ulnocarpal impingement: ulnar-shortening osteotomy with/without LT repair/reconstruction/arthrodesis
- Additional options: selective neurectomies also can be used alone or in combination with the previously mentioned interventions to augment pain relief
- Complete rupture with adjacent articular degenerative changes: proximal row carpectomy (if the proximal capitate is spared) or four-corner fusion (if the proximal lunate is spared)

In addition to the diagnostic arthroscopy, the surgeon can also perform PIN and AIN. These selective neurectomies have been shown to be effective at treating wrist instability and degenerative pathologies.[11–13] These can be performed using a longitudinal incision centered over the fourth dorsal extensor compartment between the radius and ulna proximal to the distal radioulnar joint.[11] The PIN is identified in the floor of the fourth dorsal compartment, whereas the AIN is identified after dissection through the interosseous membrane. The denervation is carried out by sectioning 1 cm of each sensory nerve, followed by a standard closure and 3 weeks of immobilization.[11–13]

Although this is rare in the chronic setting, if the LT ligament is partially torn (dorsal ligament tear with an intact volar ligament), a primary repair can be attempted as previously described.[2,5,10,16,22,26] Direct repair can be performed through a longitudinal incision over the fourth extensor compartment, creating an ulnar-based extensor retinacular flap to expose the third, fourth, and fifth extensor compartments. A PIN neurectomy is performed, followed by a ligament-sparing capsulotomy.[27] Given the close association of the intrinsic LT ligament with the radiotriquetral extrinsic ligament, it is critical to carefully dissect the capsule free of the LT ligament during the capsulotomy.[16] Inspection of the dorsal (direct) and volar (indirect with a probe) LT ligaments is performed, confirming a tear of the dorsal ligament and an intact volar ligament. The articular surfaces of the radiocarpal and midcarpal joints are also inspected for any chondral pathology. The dorsal LT ligament is then reattached to either the triquetrum or lunate using nonabsorbable suture anchors, reduced anatomically, and secured in place with 0.045 K-wires. If desired, a dorsal capsulodesis can be used to augment the repair by placing additional suture anchors on the dorsal aspects of the lunate and triquetrum to anchor the radiotriquetral ligament. The capsule, retinaculum, and skin are closed in standard fashion and the wrist is immobilized for 10 to 12 weeks.

TECHNIQUE: LUNOTRIQUETRAL RECONSTRUCTION

In cases of chronic complete (volar and dorsal) LT rupture, LT reconstruction is considered with the use of a tendon autograft or allograft. A technique using a distally based ECU graft was introduced by Reagan and colleagues[5] and later modified by Shin and Bishop[16] and Shahane and colleagues.[20] Briefly, a dorsal approach to the wrist is used from the third through fifth extensor compartments, performing a ligament-sparing capsulotomy, and exposing the LT ligament (as described previously). After LT inspection, the lunate and triquetrum are reduced anatomically and stabilized

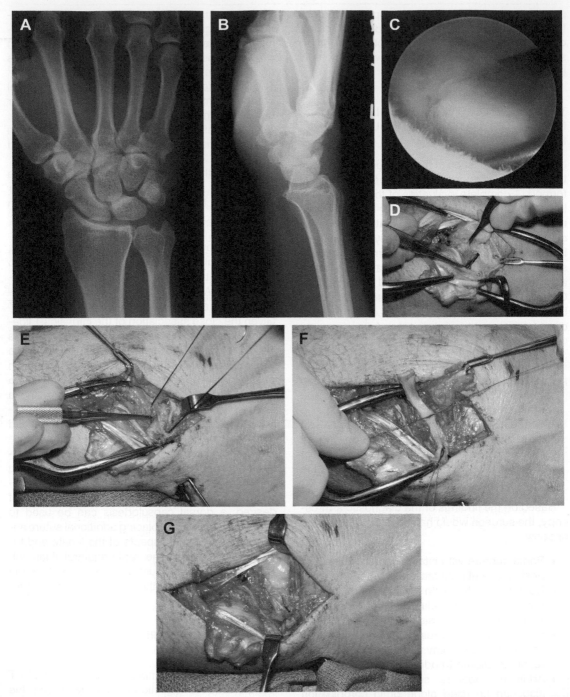

Fig. 3. Case example of a 48-year-old man with a chronic LT ligament injury. (*A* and *B*) Posteroanterior (PA) and lateral radiographs show no obvious abnormalities. He underwent arthroscopy, which showed a Geissler 3 dissociation (*C*). Open dorsal exposure of the interval revealed an irreparable lesion (*D*). Reconstruction using allograft ligament augmentation and dorsal capsule was performed. First the interval was reduced and percutaneously pinned (*E*). The ligament augmentation using cadaver dermis was attached with suture anchors (*F*) and a portion of the dorsal intercarpal ligament was anchored to the lunate (*G*). The interval was pinned for 8 weeks (*H* and *I*). The patient had good pain relief and return of function following recovery.

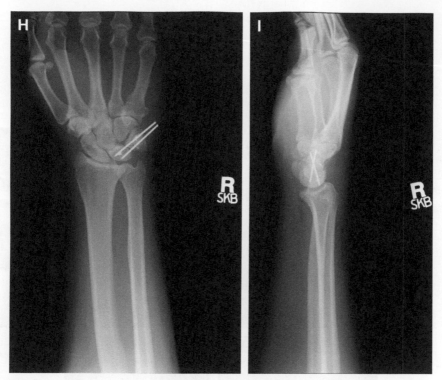

Fig. 3. (*continued*)

with extra-articular K-wires. After fluoroscopic confirmation 4- to 5-mm tunnels are drilled through the lunate and triquetrum. Next, the ECU tendon is harvested through a 2-cm transverse incision 6-cm proximal to the ulnar styloid. The ECU tendon is identified and split in half, with the radial half passed distally through the distal ECU subsheath opening. The ECU's distal attachment is left in place. The wire or suture attached to the proximal end of the tendon is then passed through the triquetral and lunate tunnels. The graft is tensioned, LT articulation is reduced, and two intra-articular K-wires are placed percutaneously to stabilize the construct. The graft is sutured back to itself and the capsule, retinaculum, and skin are closed in the usual fashion. The wrist is immobilized for 10 to 12 weeks. Alternatives to the ECU include using the dorsal intercarpal ligament and/or allograft to reconstruct the ligament (**Fig. 3**).[28]

LUNOTRIQUETRAL ARTHRODESIS

In patients with complete (dorsal and volar) LT tears, another salvage procedure is the LT arthrodesis. The wrist is approached through a dorsal longitudinal incision, exposing the dorsal wrist capsule with an ulnar-based retinacular flap. The LT joint is then exposed after a ligament-sparing capsulotomy (see previously). The LT articulation is then debrided and the cartilage is denuded using a curette or burr. After preparation of the joint surfaces, the lunate is reduced anatomically with respect to the triquetrum. Reduction is confirmed on biplanar fluoroscopy. Corticocancellous bone graft is then placed to augment the overall contact area between the two bones. The source of graft can either be autologous (local distal radius or iliac crest) or allogeneic. The lunate and triquetrum are then fixed with either K-wires, Herbert screws, or compression screws. The capsule is closed with nonabsorbable sutures, and then the retinaculum and skin are closed in the usual manner. The wrist is immobilized for 10 to 12 weeks.

ULNAR-SHORTENING OSTEOTOMY

Positive ulnar variance disrupts the biomechanics of the LT articulation, leading to abnormal stresses and potential for degenerative changes.[23,24] Furthermore, ulnocarpal impaction has been noted in up to 23% of patients following LT arthrodesis.[10] Therefore, an ulnar-shortening osteotomy is a reasonable option for isolated LT tears (**Fig. 4**). The theory behind this procedure is two-fold: correction of ulnar-positive variance helps improve wrist biomechanics; and ulnar-shortening osteotomies tension the ulnotriquetral

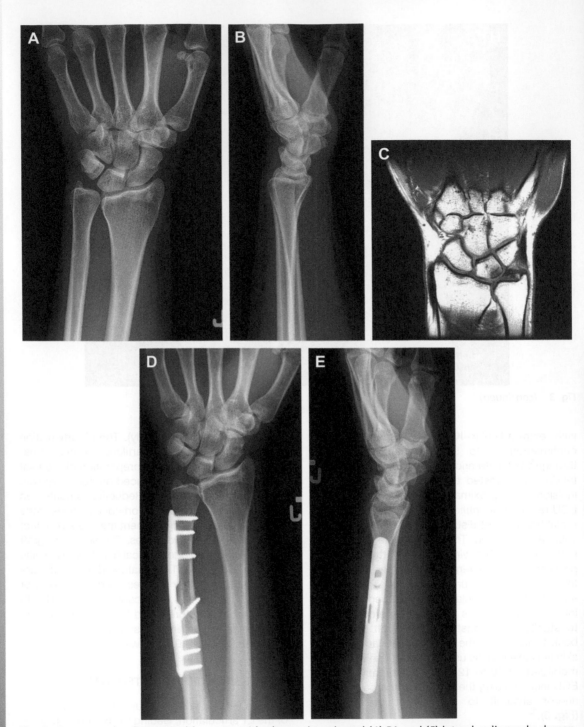

Fig. 4. Case example of 45-year-old woman with ulnar wrist pain and (A) PA and (B) lateral radiographs demonstrating positive ulnar variance. (C) T1-weighted MRI illustrates changes in the inferior portion of the LT ligament, triangular fibrocartilage complex tear, and edema changes in the lunate where it impacts the ulnar head. In addition to arthroscopy, the patient underwent ulnar-shortening osteotomy. (D) PA and (E) lateral radiographs show union of the ulna and neutral ulnar variance. The patient had good pain relief and return to function.

and ulnolunate ligaments, stabilizing the LT articulation.

This procedure can be performed using a 6- to 10-cm lateral incision 4 to 5 cm proximal to the ulnar styloid. The interval between the flexor carpi ulnaris and ECU can be used for exposure of the ulna. Minimally periosteal dissection can be performed to preserve the blood supply of the bone. After exposing the ulnar shaft, the ulna is shortened the predetermined amount based on neutral PA of the wrist. This can be done transversely or multiple systems have jigs that allow for a more precise and oblique osteotomy.[29] Fluoroscopy is helpful in confirming the appropriate amount of shortening. A compression plate is then placed either on the lateral or volar surfaces, paying close attention to AO principles of compression plating and lag screw fixation (if desired) across the osteotomy. Placement of the plate whenever possible to minimize irritation can be helpful to minimize the need for hardware removal following union. Postoperatively, the wrist and forearm are immobilized for 6 to 10 weeks.

SUMMARY

Chronic LT injuries are rare and may be challenging to diagnose. It is important to understand the varying etiologies of pain in the ulnar side of the wrist and a thorough physical examination helps clue in the diagnosis. Unfortunately, traditional imaging modalities, such as plain radiographs, are inconsistently helpful. MRI is better, but the gold standard remains diagnostic arthroscopy. Because of their chronic nature, primary surgical repair is not likely feasible. Ligament reconstruction and arthrodesis are more viable surgical options. In patients with positive ulnar variance and ulnocarpal impingement, an ulnarshortening osteotomy may be very helpful.

REFERENCES

1. Ritt MJ, Bishop AT, Berger RA, et al. Lunotriquetral ligament properties: a comparison of three anatomic subregions. J Hand Surg Am 1998;23:425–31.
2. Shin AY, Deitch MA, Sachar K, et al. Ulnar-sided wrist pain: diagnosis and treatment. Instr Course Lect 2005;54:115–28.
3. Palmer AK. Triangular fibrocartilage complex lesions: a classification. J Hand Surg Am 1989;14: 594–606.
4. Palmer AK, Werner FW. Biomechanics of the distal radioulnar joint. Clin Orthop Relat Res 1984;(275): 26–35.
5. Reagan DS, Linscheid RL, Dobyns JH. Lunotriquetral sprains. J Hand Surg Am 1984;9:502–14.
6. Kleinman WB. Diagnostic exams for ligamentous injuries. Rosemont (IL): American Society for Surgery of the Hand, Correspondence Club Newsletter; 1985. No 51.
7. Beckenbaugh RD. Accurate evaluation and management of the painful wrist following injury. An approach to carpal instability. Orthop Clin North Am 1984;15:289–306.
8. Gilula LA, Weeks PM. Post-traumatic ligamentous instabilities of the wrist. Radiology 1978;129:641–51.
9. Leon-Lopez MM, Salva-Coll G, Garcia-Elias M, et al. Role of the extensor carpi ulnaris in the stabilization of the lunotriquetral joint. An experimental study. J Hand Ther 2013;26:312–7 [quiz: 317].
10. Shin AY, Weinstein LP, Berger RA, et al. Treatment of isolated injuries of the lunotriquetral ligament. A comparison of arthrodesis, ligament reconstruction and ligament repair. J Bone Jt Surg Br 2001;83: 1023–8.
11. Berger RA. Partial denervation of the wrist: a new approach. Tech Hand Up Extrem Surg 1998;2: 25–35.
12. Hofmeister EP, Moran SL, Shin AY. Anterior and posterior interosseous neurectomy for the treatment of chronic dynamic instability of the wrist. Hand (N Y) 2006;1:63–70.
13. Weinstein LP, Berger RA. Analgesic benefit, functional outcome, and patient satisfaction after partial wrist denervation. J Hand Surg Am 2002;27:833–9.
14. Weiss AP, Sachar K, Glowacki KA. Arthroscopic debridement alone for intercarpal ligament tears. J Hand Surg Am 1997;22:344–9.
15. Westkaemper JG, Mitsionis G, Giannakopoulos PN, et al. Wrist arthroscopy for the treatment of ligament and triangular fibrocartilage complex injuries. Arthroscopy 1998;14:479–83.
16. Shin AY, Bishop AT. Treatment options for lunotriquetral dissociation. Tech Hand Up Extrem Surg 1998;2: 2–17.
17. Antti-Poika I, Hyrkas J, Virkki LM, et al. Correction of chronic lunotriquetral instability using extensor retinacular split: a retrospective study of 26 patients. Acta Orthop Belg 2007;73:451–7.
18. Omokawa S, Fujitani R, Inada Y. Dorsal radiocarpal ligament capsulodesis for chronic dynamic lunotriquetral instability. J Hand Surg Am 2009;34: 237–43.
19. Sennwald GR, Fischer M, Mondi P. Lunotriquetral arthrodesis. A controversial procedure. J Hand Surg Br 1995;20:755–60.
20. Shahane SA, Trail IA, Takwale VJ, et al. Tenodesis of the extensor carpi ulnaris for chronic, post-traumatic lunotriquetral instability. J Bone Joint Surg Br 2005; 87:1512–5.
21. Nelson DL, Manske PR, Pruitt DL, et al. Lunotriquetral arthrodesis. J Hand Surg Am 1993;18: 1113–20.

22. Kirschenbaum D, Coyle MP, Leddy JP. Chronic luno-triquetral instability: diagnosis and treatment. J Hand Surg Am 1993;18:1107–12.

23. Gupta R, Bingenheimer E, Fornalski S, et al. The effect of ulnar shortening on lunate and triquetrum motion: a cadaveric study. Clin Biomech (Bristol, Avon) 2005;20:839–45.

24. Mirza A, Mirza JB, Shin AY, et al. Isolated lunotriquetral ligament tears treated with ulnar shortening osteotomy. J Hand Surg Am 2013;38:1492–7.

25. Geissler WB, Freeland AE, Savoie FH, et al. Intracarpal soft-tissue lesions associated with an intra-articular fracture of the distal end of the radius. J Bone Joint Surg Am 1996;78:357–65.

26. Pin PG, Young VL, Gilula LA, et al. Management of chronic lunotriquetral ligament tears. J Hand Surg Am 1989;14:77–83.

27. Berger RA, Bishop AT. A fiber-splitting capsulotomy technique for dorsal exposure of the wrist. Tech Hand Up Extrem Surg 1997;1:2–10.

28. Schweizer A, Steiger R. Long-term results after repair and augmentation ligamentoplasty of rotatory subluxation of the scaphoid. J Hand Surg Am 2002; 27:674–84.

29. Rayhack JM, Gasser SI, Latta LL, et al. Precision oblique osteotomy for shortening of the ulna. J Hand Surg Am 1993;18:908–18.

Midcarpal Instability
A Comprehensive Review and Update

Timothy Niacaris, MD, PhD, Bryan W. Ming, MD,
David M. Lichtman, MD*

KEYWORDS

- Midcarpal instability • Wrist injury • Ligament • Snapping

KEY POINTS

- Midcarpal instability (MCI) has been well described as a clinical entity but the pathokinematics and pathologic anatomy continue to be poorly understood.
- MCI can be classified into intrinsic and extrinsic categories. The intrinsic category can be further subdivided into palmar, dorsal, or combined MCI instability.
- The midcarpal shift test is often diagnostic for assessment of MCI. Videofluoroscopy of the wrist can assist in diagnosis of MCI.
- Three-point splinting and proprioceptive training of dynamic wrist stabilizers (such as the extensor carpi ulnaris) can effectively manage many forms of MCI.
- The most common form of MCI is palmar MCI (PMCI). Reefing of the dorsal capsule can stabilize PMCI that persists after nonoperative management.

INTRODUCTION

Midcarpal instability (MCI) has been well described as a clinical entity but the pathokinematics and pathologic anatomy of this disorder are not fully understood. This discrepancy occurs because most theories on MCI pathomechanics and pathologic anatomy are derived from empiric clinical observations rather than quantifiable laboratory analyses. As a result, several clinical descriptors have been given to the entities resulting from the observed pathomechanics. These include the snapping wrist,[1] palmar MCI,[2] capitolunate instability pattern,[3] chronic capitolunate instability (CCI),[4] adaptive carpal instability,[5] and carpal instability nondissociative.[6] Although each of these descriptors has circumstantial evidence that suggests a specific, unique cause, they have in common

some form of altered anatomy that leads to hypermobility of the proximal row. This results in changes in the flow of normal joint reaction forces across the midcarpal joint. An understanding of this normal flow of forces is essential to understanding MCI.

WRIST BIOMECHANICS

Since the 1500s, scientists have been intrigued by the mechanics of the wrist joint. Early descriptions of the wrist by Sir Charles Bell depicted the wrist as a "composite ball and socket articulation." In the following century, several illustrative models of wrist mechanics were developed to explain carpal structure and function. Among these were Navarro's[7] columnar model, the link theory described by Gilford and colleagues,[8] which was later modified by Taleisnik and Watson,[5] and

Department of Orthopaedic Surgery, University of North Texas Health Science Center, John Peter Smith Hospital Network, 1500 South Main, Fort Worth, TX 76104, USA
* Corresponding author.
E-mail address: dlichtman@jpshealth.org

Hand Clin 31 (2015) 487–493
http://dx.doi.org/10.1016/j.hcl.2015.04.004
0749-0712/15/$ – see front matter © 2015 Elsevier Inc. All rights reserved.

hand.theclinics.com

the "slider crank" analogy envisioned by Linscheid and colleagues.[6] Their 1972 paper introduced the concepts of dorsal intercalated segment instability (DISI) and volar intercalated segment instability (VISI), further linking radiographic deformity to existing biomechanical models.

Although the carpus does behave as an intercalated link in certain pathologic circumstances, thinking of the scaphoid as a "slider crank" or the wrist as a "columnar" force model leads to confusion when trying to understand or predict the deformities and pathologic carpal interactions seen in various carpal instabilities. For this reason, the ring theory of wrist kinematics was introduced in 1981.[9] This concept envisions the carpus as 2 distinct transverse carpal rows connected by physiologic links at the scaphotrapezial (STT) and triquetrohamate (TH) joints. A key concept of the ring theory is that reciprocal motion occurs between the proximal and distal carpal rows during radial and ulnar deviation of the wrist. Each row, however, is intrinsically stable with individual components within the row moving synchronously in the same direction. In the normal wrist, radial deviation of the distal row (and hand) concentrates forces at the STT link, causing the proximal row to rotate into flexion; whereas ulnar deviation concentrates forces at the TH link, causing the proximal row to rotate into extension. External forces initiate radial and ulnar deviation but flexion and extension of the proximal row is induced and guided strictly by physiologic reactive forces acting across the radiocarpal and midcarpal joints. When the wrist is motionless, opposing joint reaction forces are balanced across the proximal row. In this balanced state, axial compression does not cause intercarpal motion or instability. Carpal instability occurs when there is a disruption of the bony or ligamentous ring within or between the proximal and distal carpal rows. In these circumstances the bony components are no longer connected, the intercarpal forces are no longer balanced, and each bony component is free to react to forces acting on it locally. Within the proximal row, this disruption leads to nonphysiologic dissociative deformities (ie, scapholunate or lunotriquetral instability) and between the 2 rows it results in MCI. Visualizing the ring model in this way, the clinically observed intercalated deformities and pathokinematic patterns are predicable based on the location of the pathologic anatomy and the locally applied force vectors.

In 1985, Palmer and colleagues[10] described the primary functional motions of the wrist to be radial deviation with extension and ulnar deviation with flexion, as in throwing a dart. This "dart thrower's motion" occurs primarily at the midcarpal joint.

Preservation of normal biomechanics within the midcarpal joint is likely critical for this motion and has important implications clinically, particularly in cases of MCI.

CLASSIFICATION OF CARPAL INSTABILITIES

Carpal instabilities can be divided into perilunate (scapholunate and lunotriquetral), midcarpal, and proximal carpal instability patterns (**Box 1**). Linscheid and colleagues[6] preferred the terms dissociative, midcarpal nondissociative, and proximal carpal nondissociative, respectively. Perilunate instabilities are caused by disruptions between discrete components of the proximal carpal row as described by Mayfield and colleagues[11] in the

---

Box 1
Classification of carpal instabilities

- Perilunate instability (carpal instability dissociative)
  - Lesser arc pattern
    - Scapholunate instability
    - Lunotriquetral instability
    - Complete perilunate dislocation
  - Greater arc pattern
    - Scaphoid fracture
      - Stable
      - Unstable (DISI)
    - Naviculocapitate syndrome
    - Transscaphoid transtriquetral perilunate dislocations
    - Variations and combinations of greater arc injury patterns
- MCI (carpal instability nondissociative)
  - Intrinsic (ligamentous laxity)
    - Palmar MCI (VISI)
    - Dorsal MCI (DISI)
    - Combined
  - Extrinsic
- Proximal carpal instability
  - Ulnar translocation of the carpus
  - Dorsal instability (after dorsal rim fracture)
  - Palmar instability (after volar rim fracture)
- Miscellaneous
  - Axial
  - Periscaphoid

1970s. These may be completely ligamentous (lesser arc) or a combination of bony and ligamentous injuries (greater arc). MCI is caused by a loss of longitudinal ligament constraints that lead to hypermobility of the proximal row relative to the distal row and radius. Proximal carpal instability occurs because of laxity of longitudinal radiocarpal and ulnocarpal ligaments, which permit translation of the proximal carpal row relative to the radius and ulna.

MCI can be further subclassified into intrinsic and extrinsic categories (**Box 2**). The extrinsic pattern is caused by structural abnormalities initiated outside the carpus. Taleisnik and Watson[5] first described this pattern in their series of MCI cases caused by malunion of the distal radius with secondary adaptive changes in the carpus. The intrinsic category of MCI is caused by pathologic anatomy within the wrist itself and is subdivided according to the direction and pathomechanics of the underlying instability. Louis and colleagues[3] and Johnson and Carrera[4] best characterized the dorsal intrinsic pattern of MCI in their articles describing the capitate lunate instability pattern (CLIP) wrist and CCI, respectively. Palmar MCI (PMCI) is the most common form of MCI seen clinically and was described by Lichtman and colleagues[9] in 1981. Apergis[12] presented cases with characteristics of both dorsal and palmar instability patterns, which may represent a more global ligamentous laxity.

DORSAL MIDCARPAL INSTABILITY

Louis and colleagues[3] described a series of patients with pain and clicking in the wrist and a dynamic dorsal subluxation of the capitate from the lunate. They postulated that dynamic laxity of the dorsal capsular ligaments (radiolunate and dorsal capitolunate) contributes to this instability and termed the entity CLIP wrist. In their study, activity modification alone resulted in relief of symptoms in 10 of 11 subjects. Johnson and Carrera[4] described 12 subjects who reported wrist pain,

weakness, and clicking following an extension injury to the wrist. Although physical examination and static radiographs are unremarkable in these wrists, dorsal capitate–displacement stress testing using fluoroscopy demonstrates dorsal subluxation of the capitate on the lunate. Additionally this maneuver recreates the clinical symptoms in these subjects. The investigators concluded that traumatic attenuation of the palmar radiocapitate ligament was the source of the symptoms. They named this pattern CCI and successfully treated it by reefing the palmar radiocapitate ligament to the radiotriquetral ligament, effectively closing the space of Poirier.

It is likely that both CLIP wrist and CCI are variants of dorsal midcarpal subluxation. Whether it is the dorsal or volar ligaments that contribute more to stability between the capitate and lunate is not known. Johnson and Carrera[4] showed that volar reefing is effective in treating dorsal midcarpal subluxation, a finding that indicates an etiologic role for the volar ligaments; however, Louis and colleagues[3] demonstrated that nonsurgical management also produces satisfactory patient outcomes.

EXTRINSIC MIDCARPAL INSTABILITY

On occasion, patients with malunion of the distal radius develop an uncomfortable wrist clunk, particularly when there is a dorsal tilt to the radius. Taleisnik and Watson[5] described 13 subjects who presented with a clunk associated with a distal radius malunion. On radiographic evaluation, the average residual dorsal tilt was 23°. The lunate was shown to migrate dorsally and tilt palmarly (VISI pattern) to compensate for fracture displacement. They described this entity as an adaptive carpus. The investigators hypothesized that the clunk is due to repetitive overload of the midcarpal ligaments. Eventually, the intact ligaments are incapable of preventing excessive translation of the capitate and permit subluxation of the midcarpal joint and clunking of the wrist with ulnar deviation. Treatment focuses on corrective osteotomy of the radius, with good results reported after realignment of the carpus.

PALMAR MIDCARPAL INSTABILITY

PMCI, the most common form of MCI, occasionally occurs after acute trauma but typically occurs in patients having universally lax ligaments. There have been reports of PMCI in patients with paraplegia following chronic overload of wrist ligaments.[13] Although symptoms are often unilateral, examination sometimes reveals bilateral laxity of

---

Box 2
Intrinsic and extrinsic categories of midcarpal instabilities

- Intrinsic
  - Palmar
  - Dorsal
  - Combined
- Extrinsic (adaptive carpus)

the midcarpal ligaments. Additionally, a more frequent presentation occurs in adolescent patients, in whom hormonal changes may contribute to ligamentous laxity. As in patients with subluxating patellae, it is prudent to avoid immediate surgery in patients with global ligamentous laxity. Adolescents with physiologically lax ligaments will most likely tighten up with time.

As described previously, MCI is due to lax ligaments (congenital, adaptive, or traumatic) between the carpal rows, resulting in poorly controlled motion of the proximal row when subjected to dynamic joint reactive forces. In the case of PMCI, the proximal row sags into volar flexion due to laxity of the volar arcuate, the dorsal radiotriquetral, and/or the periscaphoid (STT) ligaments. During ulnar deviation of the wrist from neutral, the normal joint reaction forces are not engaged and the proximal row maintains its flexed (VISI) posture well into ulnar deviation. When the TH joint is finally engaged as the wrist nears maximal ulnar deviation, the physiologic joint reaction forces are reactivated and the proximal row is forcefully rotated from VISI into its physiologic extended (DISI) posture. It is this sudden, forceful rotation that causes the catch-up clunk of PMCI.

The typical patient with PMCI is 20 to 30 years of age and has an uncomfortable clunking sensation in the wrist with activities that require twisting, squeezing, or other extreme wrist motions. Physical examination reveals ulnar-sided wrist tenderness focused at the TH joint. With the wrist unsupported, there is volar sag on the ulnar side of the wrist that can be confused with dorsal subluxation of the ulna. With active ulnar deviation there is a painful and often audible clunk with spontaneous reduction of the visible ulnar sag. Most patients can recreate this clunk without examiner assistance but, if not, the midcarpal shift test[14] can be diagnostic (**Fig. 1**). In this test, the examiner steadies the patient's pronated forearm with 1 hand while applying palmarly directed pressure with the opposite thumb on the base of the

patient's third metacarpal. This maneuver accentuates the existing palmar subluxation of the distal row and disengages the normal intercarpal contact points. The examiner then moves the wrist into ulnar deviation. As the wrist nears complete ulnar deviation, a strong clunk is felt, and often heard, as the distal row snaps back to its physiologic position. Because the clunk can occasionally be elicited in individuals with physiologically lax ligaments, the test is only considered positive when it recreates the patient's symptoms. An interesting and important corollary observation is that dorsally directed pressure on the pisiform in patients with an active clunk almost always eliminates the clunk. This is because the maneuver rotates the proximal row out of its flexed position; thereby reengaging the normal midcarpal joint contact forces. This finding has significant therapeutic implications (see later discussion).

Plain radiograph typically shows a VISI configuration on lateral views. If the wrist is supported, however, the radiograph may be normal. When carefully performed, however, videofluoroscopy is diagnostic. The wrist is studied in both the sagittal and frontal planes while the patient is recreating the clunk. If the patient cannot create the clunk actively, the midcarpal shift test should be performed under fluoroscopy using lead gloves. In the frontal plane, the examiner observes the relative motion of the bones of the proximal row, carefully ruling out any dynamic dissociative lesions. Also, in the frontal view, the examiner looks for the pathognomonic sudden jump from VISI to DISI as the wrist moves into ulnar deviation (and the distal row reduces to its physiologic position). This characteristic jump from VISI to DISI can best be seen on lateral views as the wrist approaches full ulnar deviation. As the wrist moves back to neutral, the VISI deformity once again appears on all views.

The first-line treatment of PMCI consists of nonoperative management with a focus on activity modification. On occasion, the use of passive splinting and nonsteroidal antiinflammatory drugs

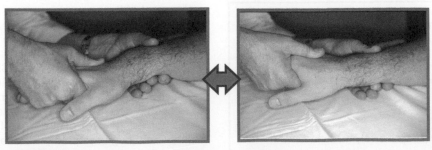

Fig. 1. Midcarpal shift test.

will fully alleviate the symptoms such that surgical management is not required. As mentioned earlier, a dorsally directed force applied through the pisiform, transmitted to the triquetrum through the pisotriquetral joint, can reduce the VISI (flexed) position of the lunate and proximal row. This effectively reestablishes physiologic midcarpal joint reactive forces and motion. Consequently, a 3-point dynamic splint that pushes up on the pisiform (**Fig. 2**) can be made to restore physiologic carpal motion in many patients. With input from a hand therapist who understands the mechanics of MCI, a form-fitting orthosis can be fashioned that permits activities of daily living without experiencing an uncomfortable clunk. In time, many patients will note an abatement of symptoms to the point that further treatment is unnecessary.

As experience has been gained in working with patients who have PMCI it has also become clear that the midcarpal clunk can be precluded by the activation of certain dynamic stabilizers of the wrist. This observation, in conjunction with recent evidence that wrist ligaments are richly endowed with proprioceptors, provides an opportunity to use proprioceptive training to aid in nonsurgical management.[15] The authors think that, in patients with wrist ligament injuries, it may be the loss of proprioception with subsequent deactivation of secondary muscle stabilizers, as much as the actual loss of structural support, that manifests as MCI. Proprioceptive training has been successfully used in the treatment of knee, shoulder, and ankle instability and research is now ongoing to help apply these concepts in MCI. As noted previously, dorsally directed pressure over the pisiform can reduce the VISI deformity in patients with MCI.[9] It is our experience that patients can be successfully taught to maintain this posture to prevent midcarpal clunking. Identifying the musculature responsible for maintaining this position of the pisiform and teaching patients how

to voluntarily reproduce this position may be the keys to helping patients preload the wrist to eliminate the subluxation and subsequent symptomatic clunk of MCI.

There are currently several surgical options for the management of PMCI. These include reefing or reconstruction of the lax ligaments (volar arcuate, dorsal radiotriquetral, or periscaphoid), limited midcarpal arthrodesis (capitolunate, TH or 4-corner), and thermal capsulorrhaphy. In 2 small studies, reefing and reconstruction of the volar arcuate ligaments were proven to be unreliable.[16] Reefing the dorsal radiotriquetral (dorsal radiocarpal) ligament has limited long-term follow-up but is the authors' preferred method of treatment of milder cases of PMCI when nonoperative management has failed.[17] The surgery is performed through a simple longitudinal incision and by reefing the dorsal capsule between the radius and proximal carpal row (**Fig. 3**). Midcarpal arthrodesis is indicated in patients who have severe PMCI that has failed nonoperative management and, possibly, prior soft tissue procedures. The authors define MCI as severe when the examiner can no longer prevent the midcarpal clunk with dorsally directed pressure on the pisiform. Although large-scale, long-term studies are lacking that compare these 2 options, it seems that the 4-corner fusion can be successful based on publications by Lichtman and colleagues[16] and by Goldfarb and colleagues.[18] In the latter study, the investigators found that 7 of 8 subjects with PMCI had good results after 4-corner fusion. These results are in contrast to those of Rao and Culver[19] who had less success (6 of 11 subjects with good results) in treating PMCI. However, they performed midcarpal fusion using TH joint arthrodesis alone. Mason and Hargreaves[20] have suggested arthroscopic thermal capsulorrhaphy as a viable option for the treatment of PMCI with all 15 wrists in their study showing improvement or resolution of symptoms after the procedure. However, no long-term results have been reported and the risks of chondrolysis, progressive capsular shrinkage, or secondary capsular insufficiency are not yet well understood.

DISCUSSION AND FUTURE DIRECTIONS

It is clear that the understanding of MCI has greatly advanced since Mouchet and Belot's[1] initial report of the snapping wrist in 1934. The past decade, in particular, has brought an increased recognition of this disorder and larger collections of treated patients. Despite this enhanced experience, the current understanding of MCI is still limited by an incomplete awareness of the complex joint

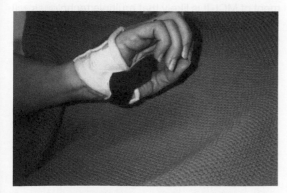

Fig. 2. Dynamic splinting for MCI.

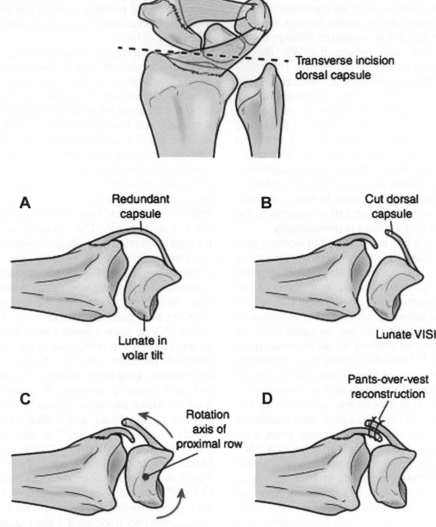

Fig. 3. Reefing of the dorsal wrist capsule in MCI.

reaction forces and soft tissue constraints that come into play during wrist motion. Several cadaveric and in vivo studies have attempted to elucidate these relationships; however, none has provided an objective, quantifiable account of what is seen clinically.

Computer-assisted modeling techniques, specifically, finite element analyses of carpal joint interrelationships,[21] is a promising area of research that can provide a more sophisticated picture of these complex relationships. These techniques can also be used to test the kinematic effects of creating both subtle and gross alterations of normal ligamentous anatomy. This is especially relevant in a system in which subtle changes in anatomy and ligament integrity could lead to profound changes in the relationship of the proximal

and distal carpal rows with wrist motion. This level of understanding will be critical to identifying both nonoperative and surgical approaches to management of MCI. It is likely that multiple techniques will need to be developed to precisely match the treatment requirements of the multiple anatomic anomalies that result in MCI.

The other area of promising research is the identification of proprioceptive mechanisms that naturally augment wrist stability. Once fully identified, patients will need to be taught how to use these mechanisms to counteract the effects of ligament laxity or injury. Based on observations described in previous sections of this article, MCI is an excellent model for testing the efficacy of proprioceptive retraining for treatment of carpal instabilities.

SUMMARY

In summary, this article attempts to clarify the current understanding of MCI by weaving together common threads of personal experience and the multiple clinical studies that have been reported over the years. Despite the relatively long interval from its first description to the present, there remains great opportunity for clinical and biomechanical research to provide evidence-based treatments for MCI.

REFERENCES

1. Mouchet A, Belot J. Poignet a'ressaut: subluxation mediocarpienne en avant. Bull Mem Soc Chir 1934;60:1243–4.
2. Lichtman DM, Gaenslen ES, Pollock GR. Midcarpal and proximal carpal instabilities. In: Lichtman DM, Alexander AH, editors. The wrist and its disorders. 2nd edition. Philadelphia: Saunders; 1997. p. 316–28.
3. Louis DS, Hankin FM, Greene TL, et al. Central carpal instability-capitate lunate instability pattern: diagnosis by dynamic displacement. Orthopedics 1984;7:1693–6.
4. Johnson RP, Carrera GF. Chronic capitolunate instability. J Bone Joint Surg Am 1986;68(8):1164–76.
5. Taleisnik J, Watson HK. Midcarpal instability caused by malunited fractures of the distal radius. J Hand Surg Am 1984;9(3):350–7.
6. Linscheid RL, Dobyns JH, Beabout JW, et al. Traumatic instability of the wrist: diagnosis, classification, and pathomechanics. J Bone Joint Surg Am 1972; 54(8):1612–32.
7. Navarro A. Luxaciones del carpo. An Fac Med 1921; 6:113–41.
8. Gilford WW, Boltan RH, Lambrinudi C. The mechanism of the wrist joint with special reference to fractures of the scaphoid. Guys Hosp Rep 1943; 92:52–9.
9. Lichtman DM, Schneider JR, Swafford AR, et al. Ulnar midcarpal instability: clinical and laboratory analysis. J Hand Surg Am 1981;6(5):515–23.
10. Palmer AK, Werner FW, Murphy D, et al. Functional wrist motion: a biomechanical study. J Hand Surg Am 1985;10(1):39–46.
11. Mayfield JK, Johnson RP, Kilcoyne RK. Carpal dislocations: pathomechanics and progressive perilunar instability. J Hand Surg Am 1980;5(3):226–41.
12. Apergis EP. The unstable capitolunate and radiolunate joints as a source of wrist pain in young women. J Hand Surg 1996;21B:501–6.
13. Schroer W, Lacey S, Frost FS, et al. Carpal instability in the weight-bearing upper extremity. J Bone Joint Surg Am 1996;78(12):1838–43.
14. Feinstein WK, Lichtman DM, Noble PC, et al. Quantitative assessment of the midcarpal shift test. J Hand Surg Am 1999;24(5):977–83.
15. Salva-Coll G, Garcia-Elias M, Hagert E. Scapholunate instability: proprioception and neuromuscular control. J Wrist Surg 2013;2(2):136–40.
16. Lichtman DM, Bruckner JD, Culp RW, et al. Palmar midcarpal instability: results of surgical reconstruction. J Hand Surg Am 1993;18(2):307–15.
17. Lichtman DM, Ming BW, Icenogle KD. Midcarpal instability. Orthopaedic Knowledge Online Journal 2014;12(3).
18. Goldfarb CA, Stern PJ, Kiefhaber TR. Palmar midcarpal instability: the results of treatment with 4-corner arthrodesis. J Hand Surg Am 2004;29(2): 258–63.
19. Rao SB, Culver JE. Triquetrohamate arthrodesis for midcarpal instability. J Hand Surg Am 1995;20(4): 583–9.
20. Mason WT, Hargreaves DG. Arthroscopic thermal capsulorrhaphy for palmar midcarpal instability. J Hand Surg Eur Vol 2007;32(4):411–6.
21. Sandow MJ, Fisher TJ, Howard CQ, et al. Unifying model of carpal mechanics based on computationally derived isometric constraints and rules-based motion – the stable central column theory. J Hand Surg Eur Vol 2013;39E(4):353–63.

Salvage Operations for Wrist Ligament Injuries with Secondary Arthrosis

Oded Ben Amotz, MD, Douglas M. Sammer, MD*

KEYWORDS

- SLAC wrist • Scapholunate • Lunotriquetral • Denervation • Four-corner arthrodesis
- Scaphoidectomy • Proximal row carpectomy

KEY POINTS

- Scapholunate advance collapse (SLAC) is a well-defined sequela of chronic scapholunate instability.
- The SLAC wrist has a predictable pattern of progression of arthrosis starting with the radioscaphoid interval and later involving the midcarpal capitolunate joint; typically, the radiolunate interval is spared.
- Wrist denervation is an established treatment of arthritis and has the advantage of simplicity and earlier recovery; denervation can also be performed in conjunction with reconstructive procedures.
- The 2 standard reconstructive options for SLAC are proximal row carpectomy and scaphoidectomy and 4-corner arthrodesis.
- Alternatives/modifications to the these traditional treatments include radial styloidectomy with and without partial wrist fusion, proximal row carpectomy with capitate resurfacing, 2-column carpal arthrodesis, and partial wrist fusion with triquetrectomy.

INTRODUCTION

The most frequently injured wrist ligament is the scapholunate interosseous ligament (SLIL), followed by the lunotriquetral interosseous ligament (LTIL). Although these ligaments may be injured in isolation, they may also represent part of a more complex ligamentous injury such as a perilunate dislocation. Wrist ligament injuries are difficult to treat successfully, and, in the case of the LTIL, the diagnosis alone can present challenges. Although the natural history of these injuries is not fully understood, untreated injuries or failed repairs often progress to carpal instability and subsequent arthrosis.

In the case of SLIL injuries, the progressive arthrosis of scapholunate ligament advanced collapse (SLAC) is well defined (**Fig. 1**).[1] Degenerative changes begin at the articulation of the radial styloid with the scaphoid (stage I), followed by involvement of the entire radioscaphoid articulation (stage II). In addition, in stage III the midcarpal (capitolunate) joint becomes involved. It is generally thought that the radiolunate joint is spared,[2] although some investigators recognize a stage IV SLAC wrist in which the radiolunate articulation is affected.[3] Other untreated ligamentous injuries, such as LTIL injuries or perilunate instability, can also progress to arthritis, although the pattern

Department of Plastic Surgery, University of Texas Southwestern Medical Center at Dallas, 1801 Inwood Road, Dallas, TX 75390, USA
* Corresponding author. University of Texas Southwestern Medical Center at Dallas, 1801 Inwood Road, Dallas, TX 75390.
E-mail address: douglas.sammer@utsouthwestern.edu

Hand Clin 31 (2015) 495–504
http://dx.doi.org/10.1016/j.hcl.2015.04.010
0749-0712/15/$ – see front matter © 2015 Elsevier Inc. All rights reserved.

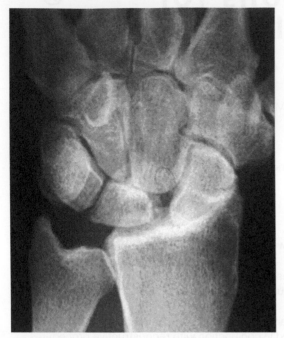

Fig. 1. Posteroanterior (PA) radiograph of the left wrist, showing a stage III SLAC wrist. Note the widened scapholunate interval, and arthrosis of the entire scaphoid fossa and capitolunate joint. As in this radiograph, the radiolunate joint is typically preserved.

of degenerative changes is not as predictable (**Figs. 2** and **3**).

In some cases, the instability and arthritis that occur as sequelae of ligamentous injuries are asymptomatic. In other cases the symptoms are mild enough that they can be managed to the patient's satisfaction with steroid injections or splinting. However, when these nonoperative modalities fail, surgical intervention is indicated. This article discusses definitive salvage operations such as

intercarpal arthrodeses and proximal row carpectomy (PRC), as well as other alternatives, such as wrist denervation and radial styloidectomy, for treating the ligamentous unstable wrist with degenerative changes.

WRIST DENERVATION PROCEDURES

The goal of wrist denervation is to divide articular nerve branches that send afferent pain signals, without affecting motor function or cutaneous sensibility. Wrist denervation was first described by Wilhelm in 1966 for the treatment of degenerative wrist arthrosis. In Wilhelm's description, articular branches of the posterior interosseous nerve (PIN), superficial sensory branch of the radial nerve, the anterior interosseous nerve (AIN), the ulnar nerve, and the median nerve are divided (10 branches in total), resulting in total wrist joint denervation. Since his original description, several investigators have studied the effectiveness of total wrist denervation, showing generally good outcomes.[4–7] A recent study of 49 wrist denervations performed for degenerative arthrosis showed pain improvement in 79% of patients, along with improvement in grip strength at 6-year follow-up.[6] Advantages of wrist denervation are that it does not adversely affect grip strength or range of motion, and does not create problems for future salvage operations. One concern is the possibility of reducing wrist proprioception, potentially resulting in neuropathic arthropathy. However, in Buck-Gramcko's[5] study of 195 complete and partial wrist denervations, no evidence of Charcot joint was found. This finding is further supported by a recent study of the effect of AIN and PIN blockade on wrist kinesthesia, in which the investigators did not find any effect on wrist proprioception.[8]

In subsequent studies, partial wrist denervation by division of the PIN, or both the PIN and AIN,

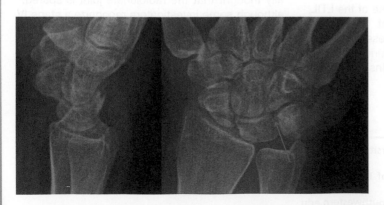

Fig. 2. Lateral (*left*) and PA (*right*) radiograph of the left wrist in a patient with a lunotriquetral ligament injury (and concomitant scapholunate injury). On lateral view, note the volar intercalated segment instability (VISI). On the PA view, note the disruption of the Gilula arc at the midcarpal joint, between the lunate and triquetrum (*red arrow*).

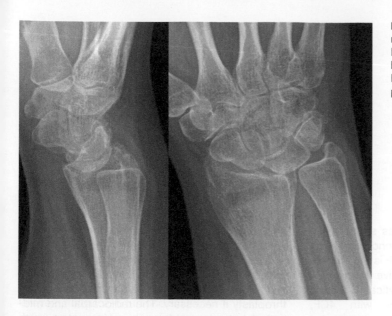

Fig. 3. Lateral (*left*) and PA (*right*) radiograph of the same wrist, 1 year later. Note the progression of instability with worsening VISI on the lateral view. On the PA view, radiocarpal and midcarpal arthrosis is seen.

has been shown to be successful in treating wrist pain.[9–11] Weinstein and Berger[9] reported 20 partial wrist denervations using a single dorsal approach to the AIN and PIN. Eighty percent of patients reported pain relief, with 45% of patients reporting increased grip strength 2.5 years postoperatively. Preoperative local anesthetic blockade of the AIN and PIN has been used to predict the success of partial wrist denervation,[10] although some investigators have found that the success of anesthetic blockade does not correlate with postoperative outcomes.[6,9]

Although the outcomes of wrist denervation have primarily been studied in patients undergoing denervation as a primary procedure, it can be applied in various clinical scenarios. Wrist denervation can be performed in patients who cannot tolerate a wrist salvage operation, or the immobilization and rehabilitation required postoperatively. It may also be performed as an adjunct to any other operation for wrist pain. In addition, it may be considered in patients who have failed the standard surgical options.

Surgical Technique: Partial Wrist Denervation

Under tourniquet control, a 4-cm longitudinal incision is made over the interosseous space between the radius and ulna. The distal end of the incision should terminate 2 cm proximal to the ulnar head. The antebrachial fascia is incised longitudinally, and the extensor tendons/muscle bellies are retracted, exposing the interosseous membrane. The PIN runs adjacent to the posterior division of the anterior interosseous artery (**Fig. 4**). A 2-cm segment of the nerve is excised. The

interosseous membrane is incised longitudinally, and the pronator quadratus muscle belly is visualized. The AIN is identified, running adjacent to the anterior interosseous artery, and a 2-cm segment of the nerve is resected. The skin is closed, and a soft bulky dressing applied. Active motion is allowed immediately.

FOUR-CORNER ARTHRODESIS VERSUS PROXIMAL ROW CARPECTOMY

The 2 standard salvage operations for SLAC wrist are scaphoidectomy with 4-corner arthrodesis (4-corner fusion [4CF]) and PRC. Both operations depend on the presence of a normal radiolunate articulation, and PRC has the further requirement of a normal head of the capitate. In the stage III SLAC wrist, in which the midcarpal joint is involved, PRC is not a viable option. However, in cases of early SLAC wrist (stage I or II), both PRC and scaphoidectomy with 4CF are reasonable alternatives. Although in general both operations result in similar outcomes, there are some differences. In a systematic review of the literature that compared the outcomes of more than 2000 scaphoidectomy with 4CFs and PRCs, both operations resulted in reliable pain relief, the wrist flexion-extension arc was in the 70° to 80° range after PRC or scaphoidectomy with 4CF, and grip strength was 70% to 75% of contralateral after either operation.[12] The postoperative arc of motion was only slightly less than preoperative motion; both operations therefore resulted in preservation of the already limited preoperative wrist motion. Note that several studies show mildly better motion after PRC than after scaphoidectomy with

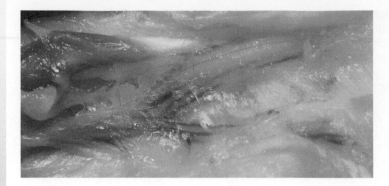

Fig. 4. The PIN (*dashed line*) is seen adjacent to the posterior division of the anterior interosseous artery.

4CF,[1,13–17] although not all studies support this distinction.[18,19] One clear difference between PRC and scaphoidectomy with 4CF is the complication rate needed for postoperative immobilization: complications were significantly more common after scaphoidectomy with 4CF, including nonunion, delayed union, and hardware-related problems, and the period of immobilization is greater for scaphoidectomy with 4CF.[12] In patients who cannot tolerate an extended period of wrist immobilization, or in heavy smokers in whom nonunion is a concern, PRC may be preferred.

Because the articulation of the capitate head with the radius is not completely congruent, progressive degenerative changes can develop at this location after PRC. However, in a 20-year follow-up study of PRC in 16 wrists, there was no correlation between patient outcomes and radiographic progression of arthritis.[20] However, patient age did correlate with outcomes, and a higher ultimate failure rate requiring conversion to total wrist arthrodesis was seen in patients younger than 40 years of age at the time of PRC. Because of this, scaphoidectomy with 4CF may be preferable in young patients.

Surgical Technique: Proximal Row Carpectomy

A longitudinal midline incision is made on the dorsal wrist in line with the third ray. Skin flaps are elevated at the level of the extensor retinaculum, keeping veins and sensory nerves within the skin flaps. The extensor retinaculum is incised along the course of the extensor pollicis longus (EPL) tendon, and the EPL is transposed radially. Retinacular flaps are elevated into the fifth compartment ulnarly, and into the second compartment radially, and the extensor tendons are retracted. The PIN is identified on the radial side of the floor of the fourth extensor compartment, adjacent to the posterior division of the anterior interosseous

neurectomy is performed as described earlier. A wrist capsulotomy is performed and the carpus exposed. The authors prefer to use a proximally based inverted U-shaped capsulotomy. In this way, the capsule may be used for interposition arthroplasty if necessary. The radiocarpal and midcarpal articular surfaces are inspected, with careful attention paid to the lunate fossa and the head of the capitate, and suitability for PRC is confirmed. The scaphoid, lunate, and triquetrum are removed, which is facilitated by dividing the SLIL and LTIL ligaments, followed by removal of each bone with a rongeur. Radiographs are taken to confirm complete removal of the proximal carpal row. It is important to carefully preserve the volar radiocarpal ligaments, in particular the radioscaphocapitate ligament, to prevent postoperative ulnar carpal translocation. The head of the capitate is seated into the lunate fossa (**Fig. 5**). The wrist is

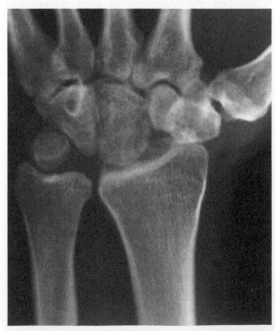

Fig. 5. PA radiograph of the left wrist, showing a PRC.

then passively ranged to confirm that there is no impingement on the radial styloid during radial deviation. If impingement occurs, a radial styloidectomy is performed as described later. Temporary pinning of the radius and capitate is unnecessary. A layered closure is performed, including capsule, retinaculum (with the EPL left transposed), and skin. A wrist splint is applied. Motion may begin 2 to 4 weeks postoperatively. Weight-bearing restrictions are removed at 3 months.

Surgical Technique: Scaphoidectomy with 4-Corner Arthrodesis

A dorsal wrist exposure is performed as described earlier. A ligament-sparing capsulotomy is performed, exposing the carpus. The articular surfaces are evaluated, confirming that the radiolunate articular surfaces are preserved. The scaphoid is removed piecemeal with an osteotome and rongeur. Care is taken to preserve the radioscaphocapitate ligament. Next, the articular surfaces are prepared for arthrodesis, including the distal surface of the lunate and triquetrum, and proximal surface of the capitate and hamate. Cartilage and subchondral bone are removed, exposing cancellous bone. On the convex surfaces, this is easily accomplished with a rongeur. Preparation of the concave surfaces is facilitated by the use of a high-speed burr. The lunotriquetral articulation is also prepared with a burr, taking care to preserve the LTIL in order to prevent bone graft from extruding into the radiocarpal joint. In addition, the capitohamate joint is prepared with a rongeur or burr. After the articular surfaces are prepared, cancellous autograft, which can be harvested from the distal radius, is packed into the fusion site. Next, carpal alignment corrected. The wrist is flexed, bringing the lunate out of its extended position and into colinearity with the radius. A temporary 0.062 Kirschner wire (K-wire) is passed from dorsal radius into the lunate, securing the lunate in neutral alignment. If the arthrodesis is performed with the lunate extended, wrist flexion is maintained, but at the expense of a loss of wrist extension.[21] Next, the midcarpal joint is reduced. Two temporary K-wires are passed across the midcarpal joint, keeping the capitate colinear with the lunate. The radiolunate K-wire is now removed and the temporary midcarpal K-wires maintain carpal reduction while fixation is performed. Fixation may be performed with K-wires, headless compression screws, staples, or a dorsal plate. The authors prefer to use cannulated headless compression screws. Several screw configurations have been described, but the authors prefer 1 longitudinal screw across

the capitolunate joint, 1 longitudinal screw across the triquetrohamate joint, and an optional oblique screw between triquetrum and capitate (**Fig. 6**). If a dorsal circular plate is used (**Fig. 7**), care must be taken to adequately ream a circular trough for the plate so that it does not sit proudly, and care must be taken to place the plate distally enough. Failure to do either of these can result in dorsal impingement of the plate with the radius during extension. In addition, care must be taken to avoid an excessively long triquetral screw, which can result in pisotriquetral joint penetration and ulnar-sided wrist pain. After placement of the triquetral screw, a supinated lateral view that profiles the pisotriquetral joint determines whether the screw length is appropriate. **Fig. 8** shows the triquetral screw and the pisotriquetral joint on postoperative computed tomography (CT) images. After fixation is completed, the wrist is passively ranged, and, if there is impingement at the radial styloid, a

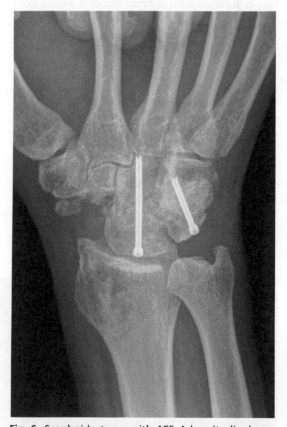

Fig. 6. Scaphoidectomy with 4CF. A longitudinal cannulated headless compression screw is advanced across the capitolunate and triquetrum-hamate joints. An oblique third screw from triquetrum to hamate is optional. Note the solid union between the 4 bones, with the exception of a portion of the lunotriquetral joint.

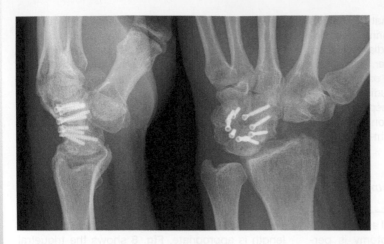

Fig. 7. Lateral (*left*) and PA (*right*) radiographs of a scaphoidectomy with 4CF performed with a dorsal circular plate. The radiolucent plate is made of polyether ether ketone, allowing improved visualization of the fusion site on radiographs. A radial styloidectomy has been performed.

styloidectomy is performed. The wound is closed as described earlier, and a wrist splint is applied. At 2 weeks postoperatively, sutures are removed and a short-arm cast is applied. Cast immobilization is continued for a minimum of 6 weeks from the time of surgery, and until bony union occurs. The authors prefer to obtain a CT scan to confirm union before allowing wrist motion.

OTHER ALTERNATIVES TO PROXIMAL ROW CARPECTOMY AND SCAPHOIDECTOMY WITH 4-CORNER FUSION
Radial Styloidectomy

Another option for stage I SLAC wrists, in which degenerative changes are restricted to the radial styloid, is radial styloidectomy. This option should be reserved for patients in whom pain is localized to the area of arthrosis at the styloid, and who are not tender over the proximal portion of the radioscaphoid joint or at the scapholunate interval. In these select patients, radial styloidectomy provides pain relief, but it does not alter the progression of degenerative changes, which may become a source of pain in the future. Care must be taken not to disrupt the origin of the volar radiocarpal ligaments, the most vulnerable of which is the radioscaphocapitate ligament. Biomechanical studies suggest that resection of more than 4 mm results in an increased risk of carpal instability.[22] Radial styloid is typically performed with an open incision over the radial styloid, although it can be performed arthroscopically as well.[23]

Scaphocapitolunate Arthrodesis with Radial Styloidectomy

Another option that has been described for stage I SLAC wrist is scaphocapitolunate arthrodesis with radial styloidectomy.[24–27] The styloidectomy addresses the arthritic articulation, and fusion of the scaphoid, capitate, and lunate corrects the

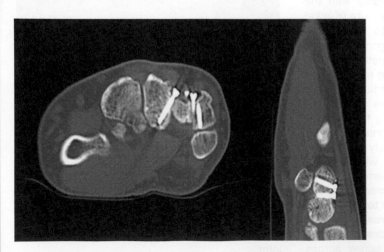

Fig. 8. Axial (*left*) and sagittal (*right*) computed tomography images show the pisotriquetral joint (*red arrows*), which can be at risk for screw impingement if the triquetral screw is excessively long.

midcarpal and scapholunate instability, thereby preventing progression of the SLAC wrist. Although the authors reserve this operation for stage I SLAC wrist, proponents note that even in stage II and III SLAC wrists, the radioscaphoid arthritis is often limited to the dorsal aspect of the scaphoid fossa and the volar surface of the flexed scaphoid. When the scaphoid is reduced, the contacting articulating surfaces are preserved, making scaphocapitolunate arthrodesis feasible in many cases of stage II or III SLAC wrist.[24] One theoretic advantage of this procedure compared with scaphoidectomy with 4CF or PRC is that it maintains a larger articular surface area at the radiocarpal joint, and distributes load more evenly. In 2012, Klausmeyer and Fernandez[24] and Klausmeyer and colleagues[28] reported the results of 20 patients at an average of 4.6 years postoperatively. Thirteen of 20 patients were pain free, and all experienced a reduction in pain. The mean flexion-extension arc was 70°, which is similar to what is expected after PRC or scaphoidectomy with 4CF.

Capitolunate Arthrodesis with and Without Triquetrum Excision

Numerous variations of the standard scaphoidectomy with 4CF have been described; most notably scaphoid excision and isolated arthrodesis of the capitolunate joint.[29] Inclusion of the triquetrum and hamate in the fusion mass is not necessary as long a solid union occurs between the capitate and lunate. Long-term outcomes are similar to those for scaphoidectomy with 4CF.[29] Although prior studies showed a higher incidence of nonunion and complications when comparing scaphoidectomy with capitolunate arthrodesis to scaphoidectomy with 4CF (35% vs 4% respectively),[30] the advent of cannulated headless compression screws and specialized staples allows predictable union of capitolunate arthrodeses. The authors prefer to use 2 cannulated headless compression screws for capitolunate arthrodesis (**Fig. 9**). As an additional alternative, the triquetrum can be excised along with the scaphoid when performing capitolunate arthrodesis (**Fig. 10**). Triquetrum excision has been shown to improve motion in cadaveric studies,[31] although its effect in vivo is not clear.

Bicolumnar Arthrodesis

Scaphoidectomy with bicolumnar arthrodesis is a modification of the standard 4CF in which a combined arthrodesis of the capitolunate and triquetrum-hamate joints is performed, without arthrodesis of the lunotriquetral joint or

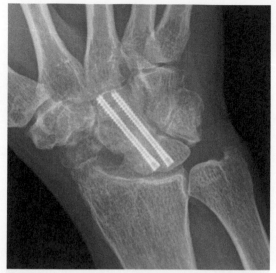

Fig. 9. PA wrist radiograph showing scaphoidectomy with isolated capitolunate arthrodesis using 2 cannulated headless compression screws.

capitohamate joint (**Fig. 11**). Because almost no motion occurs at the capitohamate joint, the entire bicolumnar arthrodesis moves as a stable unit. Outcomes are comparable with those reported for scaphoidectomy with 4CF or scaphoidectomy with capitolunate arthrodesis.[32–34]

Proximal Row Carpectomy with Osteochondral Resurfacing

Classically, PRC is contraindicated if there is arthritis involving the head of the capitate. If this is the case, scaphoidectomy with 4CF is the most reasonable operation. However, alternatives have been described that allow PRC to be performed in this setting. Tang and Imbriglia[35]

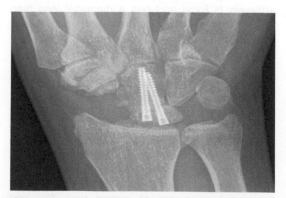

Fig. 10. PA wrist radiograph showing scaphoidectomy with isolated capitolunate arthrodesis, along with triquetrum excision, with the goal of maximizing wrist motion.

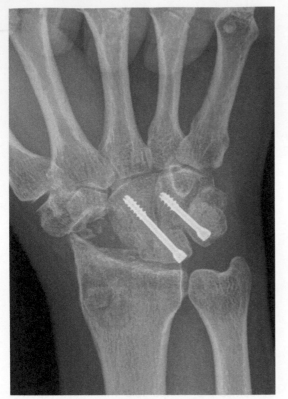

Fig. 11. PA wrist radiograph showing scaphoidectomy with bicolumnar intercarpal arthrodesis. Arthrodesis of the capitolunate joint and triquetrum-hamate joint has been performed. Note the preservation of the capitohamate and lunotriquetral joints.

described osteochondral resurfacing for capitate arthrosis when performing a PRC. The osteochondral resurfacing graft is obtained from the normal articular surfaces of the resected carpal bones. The investigators recommended osteochondral resurfacing of the capitate head if the area of arthrosis is focal and has a diameter less than 10 mm. First, the site of arthrosis is prepared using a sizer from the osteochondral autograft transfer system (OATS; Arthrex, Inc, Naples, FL). A guide pin is drilled into the area of chondrosis, and then a cannulated reamer is drilled over the guidewire to a depth of 10 mm. Next, a donor harvester is used to obtain the graft, which is then inserted into the capitate, until the cartilage is flush. The investigators reported the results 8 patients who underwent PRC in the setting of arthritis of the capitate head using this technique. Postoperatively, at an average of 18 months, the flexion-extension arc of motion was 75°, and grip strength was 62% of contralateral. Seven patients described their postoperative pain as mild to none.

Proximal Row Carpectomy with Capsular Interposition

An alternative solution to the problem of capitate head arthrosis discussed earlier is to perform the PRC with a capsular interposition.[36–40] A standard dorsal approach to the wrist is performed. The capsulotomy is made by creating a U-shaped capsular flap, based at the radiocarpal joint, and extending to the second to the fourth carpometacarpal joints. After removing the proximal carpal row, the dorsal capsular flap is turned down over the radius articular surface and sutured to the volar wrist capsule, providing a thick layer of interposed tissue between the capitate head and the lunate fossa. In a study of this technique on 8 wrists, patients had a decrease in 5-point visual analog scale pain scores from 3 to 0.8 at 41 months postoperatively. The postoperative flexion-extension arc was 72°, and grip strength was 67% of contralateral.[40] Other investigators recommend a more aggressive modification of this operation, in which capitate leveling is performed (ie, resection of the proximal end of the capitate head and hamate) along with capsular flap interposition to create a broad pseudarthrosis, and they report similar outcomes.[36,39]

SUMMARY

SLAC wrist is a sequela of chronic scapholunate instability and can result in significant wrist pain and dysfunction. When conservative measures fail, operative treatments are often used. Denervation procedures can be used to relieve pain. They are simpler than reconstructive procedures and have a more rapid postoperative recovery. The most common reconstructive procedures include PRC and scaphoidectomy and 4-corner arthrodesis. The PRC is not indicated in end-stage SLAC disease. When successful, both have been shown to provide good pain relief and adequate function. Newer alternatives/adaptations to these traditional treatments, including triquetrectomy, 2-column arthrodesis, PRC with capitate resurfacing, and radial styloidectomy with and without partial wrist fusion, have also been described.

REFERENCES

1. Krakauer JD, Bishop AT, Cooney WP. Surgical treatment of scapholunate advanced collapse. J Hand Surg 1994;19(5):751–9.
2. Watson HK, Ballet FL. The SLAC wrist: scapholunate advanced collapse pattern of degenerative arthritis. J Hand Surg 1984;9(3):358–65.
3. Zinberg EM, Chi Y. Proximal row carpectomy versus scaphoid excision and intercarpal arthrodesis:

intraoperative assessment and procedure selection. J Hand Surg 2014;39(6):1055–62.

4. Geldmacher J, Legal HR, Brug E. Results of denervation of the wrist and wrist joint by Wilhelm's method. Hand 1972;4(1):57–9.

5. Buck-Gramcko D. Denervation of the wrist joint. J Hand Surg 1977;2(1):54–61.

6. Braga-Silva J, Roman JA, Padoin AV. Wrist denervation for painful conditions of the wrist. J Hand Surg 2011;36(6):961–6.

7. Ekerot L, Holmberg J, Eiken O. Denervation of the wrist. Scand J Plast Reconstr Surg 1983;17(2):155–7.

8. Gay A, Harbst K, Hansen DK, et al. Effect of partial wrist denervation on wrist kinesthesia: wrist denervation does not impair proprioception. J Hand Surg 2011;36(11):1774–9.

9. Berger RA. Partial denervation of the wrist: a new approach. Tech Hand Up Extrem Surg 1998;2(1):25–35.

10. Dellon AL. Partial joint denervation I: wrist, shoulder, and elbow. Plast Reconstr Surg 2009;123(1):197–207.

11. Dellon AL. Partial dorsal wrist denervation: resection of the distal posterior interosseous nerve. J Hand Surg 1985;10(4):527–33.

12. Mulford JS, Ceulemans LJ, Nam D, et al. Proximal row carpectomy vs four corner fusion for scapholunate (Slac) or scaphoid nonunion advanced collapse (Snac) wrists: a systematic review of outcomes. J Hand Surg Eur Vol 2009;34(2):256–63.

13. Berkhout MJ, Bachour Y, Zheng KH, et al. Four-corner arthrodesis versus proximal row carpectomy: a retrospective study with a mean follow-up of 17 years. J Hand Surg 2015. [Epub ahead of print].

14. Cohen MS, Kozin SH. Degenerative arthritis of the wrist: proximal row carpectomy versus scaphoid excision and four-corner arthrodesis. J Hand Surg 2001;26(1):94–104.

15. Dacho AK, Baumeister S, Germann G, et al. Comparison of proximal row carpectomy and midcarpal arthrodesis for the treatment of scaphoid nonunion advanced collapse (SNAC-wrist) and scapholunate advanced collapse (SLAC-wrist) in stage II. J Plast Reconstr Aesthet Surg 2008;61(10):1210–8.

16. Tomaino MM, Miller RJ, Cole I, et al. Scapholunate advanced collapse wrist: proximal row carpectomy or limited wrist arthrodesis with scaphoid excision? J Hand Surg 1994;19(1):134–42.

17. Wyrick JD, Stern PJ, Kiefhaber TR. Motion-preserving procedures in the treatment of scapholunate advanced collapse wrist: proximal row carpectomy versus four-corner arthrodesis. J Hand Surg 1995;20(6):965–70.

18. De Smet L, Degreef I, Robijns F, et al. Salvage procedures for degenerative osteoarthritis of the wrist due to advanced carpal collapse. Acta Orthop Belg 2006;72(5):535–40.

19. Vanhove W, De Vil J, Van Seymortier P, et al. Proximal row carpectomy versus four-corner arthrodesis as a treatment for SLAC (scapholunate advanced collapse) wrist. J Hand Surg Eur Vol 2008;33(2):118–25.

20. Wall LB, Didonna ML, Kiefhaber TR, et al. Proximal row carpectomy: minimum 20-year follow-up. J Hand Surg 2013;38(8):1498–504.

21. De Carli P, Donndorff AG, Alfie VA, et al. Four-corner arthrodesis: influence of the position of the lunate on postoperative wrist motion: a cadaveric study. J Hand Surg 2007;32(9):1356–62.

22. Nakamura T, Cooney WP 3rd, Lui WH, et al. Radial styloidectomy: a biomechanical study on stability of the wrist joint. J Hand Surg 2001;26(1):85–93.

23. Yao J, Osterman AL. Arthroscopic techniques for wrist arthritis (radial styloidectomy and proximal pole hamate excisions). Hand Clin 2005;21(4):519–26.

24. Klausmeyer M, Fernandez D. Scaphocapitolunate arthrodesis and radial styloidectomy: a treatment option for posttraumatic degenerative wrist disease. J Wrist Surg 2012;1(2):115–22.

25. Rotman MB, Manske PR, Pruitt DL, et al. Scaphocapitolunate arthrodesis. J Hand Surg 1993;18(1):26–33.

26. Simmen BR, Bloch HR. Partial arthrodesis of the carpal bones in advanced carpal collapse in chronic scapholunar instability and following scaphoid pseudoarthrosis. Orthopade 1993;22(1):79–85 [in German].

27. Viegas SF. Limited arthrodesis for scaphoid nonunion. J Hand Surg 1994;19(1):127–33.

28. Klausmeyer MA, Fernandez DL, Caloia M. Scaphocapitolunate arthrodesis and radial styloidectomy for posttraumatic degenerative wrist disease. J Wrist Surg 2012;1(1):47–54.

29. Ferreres A, Garcia-Elias M, Plaza R. Long-term results of lunocapitate arthrodesis with scaphoid excision for SLAC and SNAC wrists. J Hand Surg Eur Vol 2009;34(5):603–8.

30. Siegel JM, Ruby LK. A critical look at intercarpal arthrodesis: review of the literature. J Hand Surg 1996;21(4):717–23.

31. Bain GI, Sood A, Ashwood N, et al. Effect of scaphoid and triquetrum excision after limited stabilisation on cadaver wrist movement. J Hand Surg Eur Vol 2009;34(5):614–7.

32. Draeger RW, Bynum DK Jr, Schaffer A, et al. Bicolumnar intercarpal arthrodesis: minimum 2-year follow-up. J Hand Surg 2014;39(5):888–94.

33. Mahmoud M, El Shafie S. Bicolumnar fusion for scaphoid nonunion advanced collapse without bone grafting. Tech Hand Up Extrem Surg 2012;16(2):80–5.

34. Wang ML, Bednar JM. Lunatocapitate and triquetrohamate arthrodeses for degenerative arthritis of the wrist. J Hand Surg 2012;37(6):1136–41.

35. Tang P, Imbriglia JE. Osteochondral resurfacing (OCRPRC) for capitate chondrosis in proximal row carpectomy. J Hand Surg 2007;32(9):1334–42.

36. Placzek JD, Boyer MI, Raaii F, et al. Proximal row carpectomy with capitate resection and capsular interposition for treatment of scapholunate advanced collapse. Orthopedics 2008;31(1):75.

37. Diao E, Andrews A, Beall M. Proximal row carpectomy. Hand Clin 2005;21(4):553–9.

38. Eaton RG. Proximal row carpectomy and soft tissue interposition arthroplasty. Tech Hand Up Extrem Surg 1997;1(4):248–54.

39. Salomon GD, Eaton RG. Proximal row carpectomy with partial capitate resection. J Hand Surg 1996;21(1):2–8.

40. Kwon BC, Choi SJ, Shin J, et al. Proximal row carpectomy with capsular interposition arthroplasty for advanced arthritis of the wrist. J Bone Joint Surg Br 2009;91(12):1601–6.

Index

Note: Page numbers of article titles are in **boldface** type.

Hand Clin 31 (2015) 505–507
http://dx.doi.org/10.1016/S0749-0712(15)00063-3
0749-0712/15/$ – see front matter © 2015 Elsevier Inc. All rights reserved.

hand.theclinics.com

Moving?

Make sure your subscription moves with you!

To notify us of your new address, find your **Clinics Account Number** (located on your mailing label above your name), and contact customer service at:

Email: journalscustomerservice-usa@elsevier.com

800-654-2452 (subscribers in the U.S. & Canada)
314-447-8871 (subscribers outside of the U.S. & Canada)

Fax number: 314-447-8029

**Elsevier Health Sciences Division
Subscription Customer Service
3251 Riverport Lane
Maryland Heights, MO 63043**

*To ensure uninterrupted delivery of your subscription, please notify us at least 4 weeks in advance of move.

Moving?

Make sure your subscription moves with you!

To notify us of your new address, find your Clinics Account Number (located on your mailing label above your name), and contact customer service at:

Email: journalscustomerservice-usa@elsevier.com

800-654-2452 (subscribers in the U.S. & Canada)
314-447-8871 (subscribers outside of the U.S. & Canada)

Fax number: 314-447-8029

Elsevier Health Sciences Division
Subscription Customer Service
3251 Riverport Lane
Maryland Heights, MO 63043

Printed and bound by CPI Group (UK) Ltd, Croydon, CR0 4YY

03/10/2024

01040382-0006